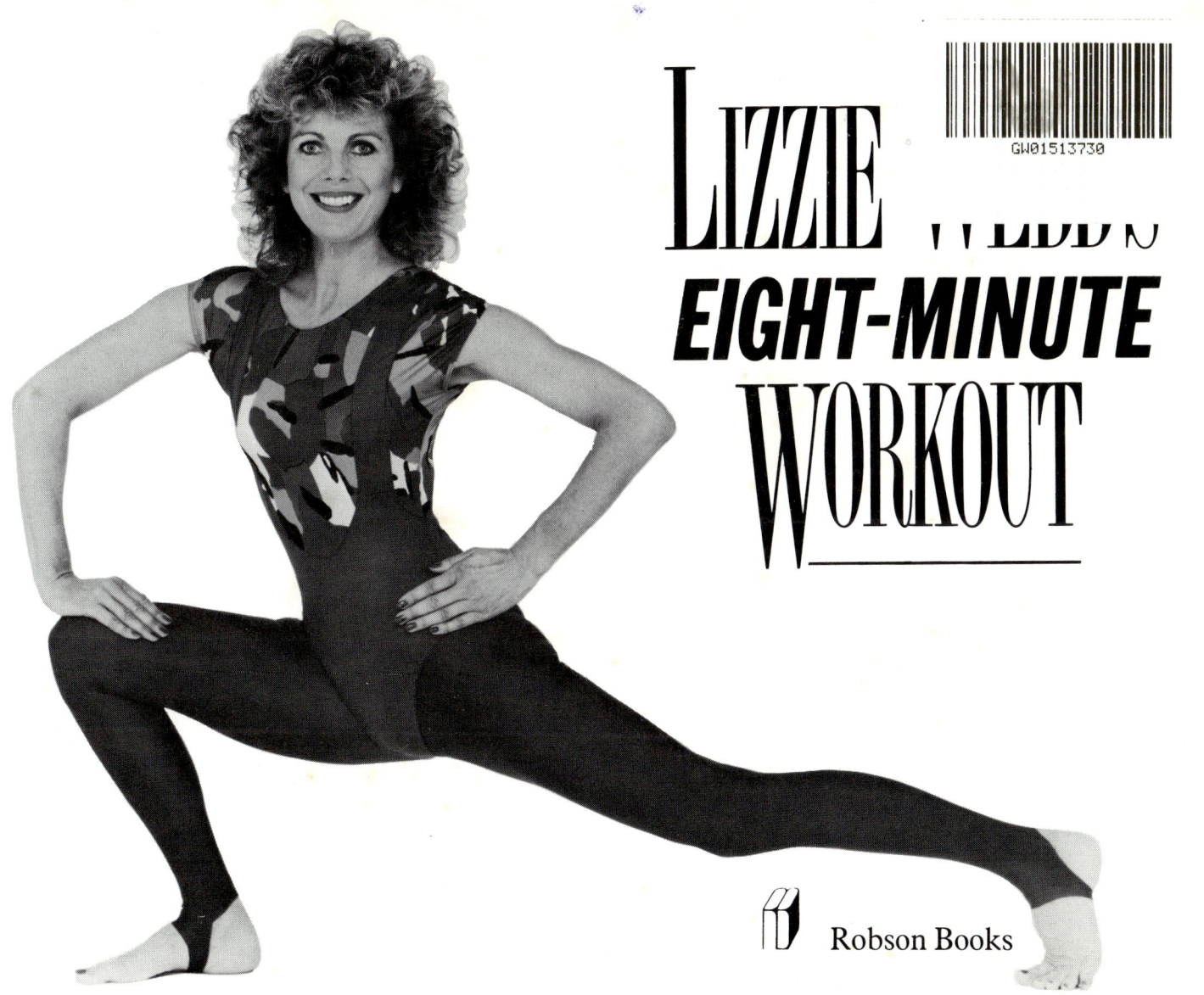

LIZZIE WEBB'S EIGHT-MINUTE WORKOUT

Robson Books

First published in Great Britain in 1991
by Robson Books Ltd, Bolsover House,
5-6 Clipstone Street, London W1P 7EB

Copyright © 1991 Lizzie Webb
The right of Lizzie Webb to be identified as
author of this work has been asserted by her
in accordance with the Copyright, Designs
and Patents Act 1988

British Library Cataloguing in Publication Data
Webb, Lizzie
   Lizzie Webb's eight-minute workouts.
   1. Physical fitness: Exercises (Movements)
   I. Title
   613.71

ISBN 0-86051-726-8

Photographs by Harry Ormesher

Every care has been taken in preparing the
exercises in this book, but readers should have
regard to their age and state of health before
following them. If you are in doubt about their
suitability for you, consult your medical advisor,
as no responsibility can be accepted by the
author or publishers.

All rights reserved. No part of this publication
may be reproduced, stored in a retrieval system,
or transmitted in any form or by any means,
electronic, mechanical, photocopying, recording
or otherwise, without the prior permission in
writing of the publishers.

Typeset by Rowland Phototypesetting Ltd,
Bury St Edmunds, Suffolk
Printed in Great Britain by
Butler & Tanner Ltd, Frome and London

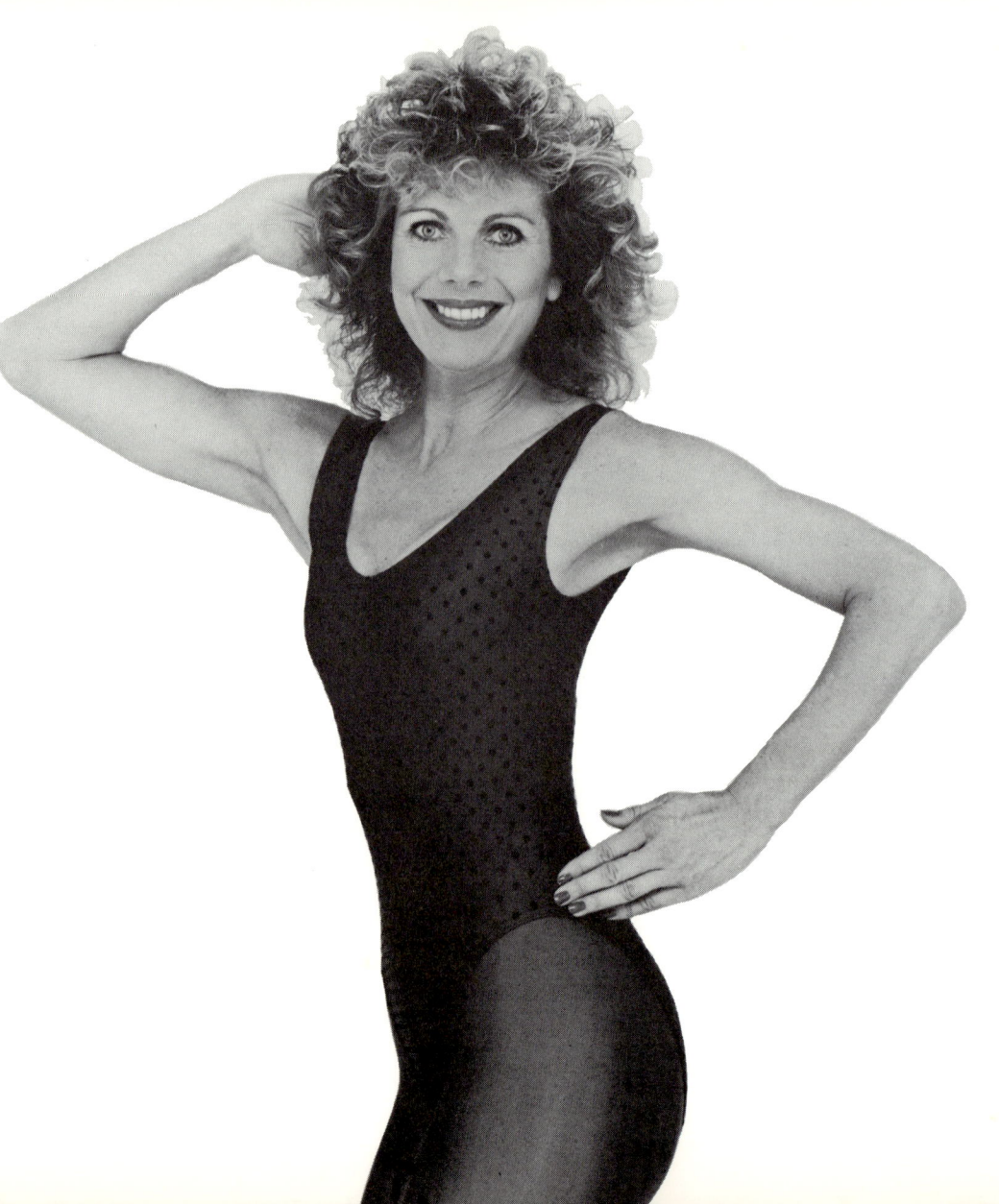

Contents

Introduction	5
The Dos and Don'ts of Exercise	7
How Fit Are You?	13
Progress Chart Jan–June	17
Monday	18
Warm Up	18
Waist	22
Tummy Stage I	26
Hips, Thighs and Bottom Stage I	30
Tuesday	34
Warm Up	34
Postural Problems	38
Back	40
Facial Exercises	44
Hips, Thighs and Bottom Stage II	48
Wednesday	52
Warm Up	52
Chair Exercises	56
Arms and Shoulders	60
Hips, Thighs and Bottom Stage III	64
Thursday	68
Stamina Day	68
Friday	84
Warm Up	84
Pop Dance	88
Leg Exercises Stage I	92
Tummy Stage II	96
Saturday	100
Warm Up	100
Hips, Thighs and Bottom Stage III	104
Leg Exercises Stage I	108
Pop Dance	112
Sunday	116
Warm Up	116
Chair Exercises	120
Leg Exercises Stage II	124
So How Are You Doing?	128
Progress Chart Jul–Dec	133

Introduction

You are born with one body — your working machine — and it's down to you to take care of it.

These eight-minute workouts — one devised for each day of the week — will help you stay fit, energetic and in shape in the 1990s. Our pace of life is hectic and stressful and it isn't always easy to re-energize to face another day. The fact is that exercise can help you do just that: with the help of these workouts you will soon see the benefit of regular daily exercise.

The enormous variety to be found in this book means that you will never become bored. Neither will you find it too much of a strain or uphill battle because all these exercises can be easily fitted into your daily routine. You can do them anywhere — just find enough space in your lounge, bedroom or even hotel room — and at any time. To begin with, your daily workout might take longer as you learn the exercises. Go at your own pace and find your own rhythm. On Thursday the workout sequence is designed to build up your stamina and exercise the cardiovascular system. This sequence will take longer than eight minutes — but then your heart is worth taking care of!

The illustrations are designed to be a 'mirror image', thus, with the book in front of you, you can read the text and see exactly what I mean by looking at the pictures — I'll be your fitness partner on the road to a better body!

Doctors recommend that we do twenty minutes' exercise three times per week to stay in good health. Why not try eight minutes seven times per week and make sure the doctor *stays* away?

Happy exercising!

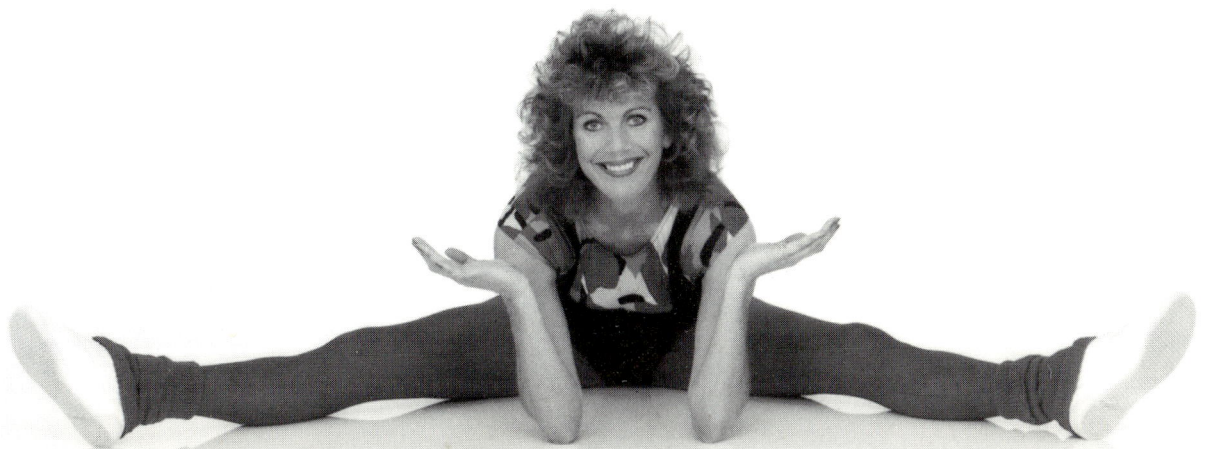

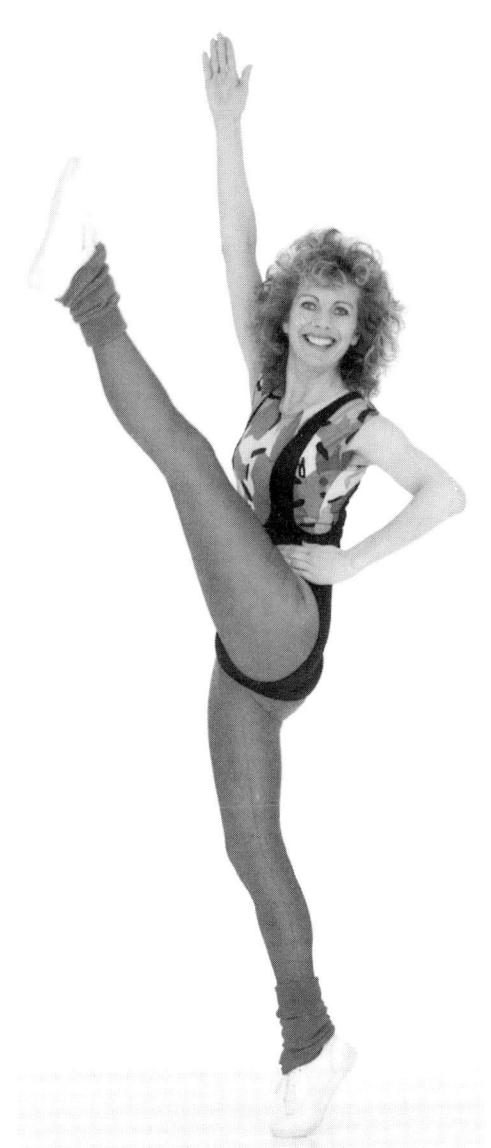

The Dos and Don'ts of Exercise

THE BASICS

Before you begin this exercise programme here are some reminders:

- Wear comfortable, loose clothing. You don't have to wear leotards and tights — leisure wear and tracksuits are ideal. But remember: what you choose to wear is psychologically important. You should *feel* good both at the start and finish of your workout, so wear colours that make you feel bright and confident. Your clothes should not restrict your movement, but neither should they be too baggy — loose folds can cause accidents by trapping arms and legs.
- Your muscles need to be warm before you begin, so make sure the room is warm, draught free and well ventilated.
- Because these are not fast aerobic workouts you do not need to wear shoes, you can exercise in bare feet, the choice is yours (indeed floor exercises can be easier in bare feet). If you do wear trainers, they should be a comfortable fit with good support.
- Don't eat or drink an hour before exercising. At the end of your workout don't have ice added to a cold drink, the temperature change is too extreme for your body. Also, make sure you keep warm after your exercise programme, particularly in winter.
- Exercise shouldn't hurt. At long last the dangerous 'no pain, no gain' principle has been abandoned, so always STOP if you feel uncomfortable twinges, any muscle trembling or shaking, gripping pains. There is a difference between all these and the general ache felt when restarting exercise after a long, inactive period.

Listen to your body, the signals mentioned above are warnings. Your body will get stronger and shaplier by you patiently increasing the amount of exercise you do, not by pushing through pain that could be caused by unnatural body movements or sheer overstress.

THE DOS AND DON'TS OF EXERCISE

LET'S MAKE A START

Never forget that you are exercising to take better care of your body, not to punish it. So, if you can't achieve any position illustrated in this book, view it as a goal, something to achieve with regular exercise.

These are the correct (and incorrect) positions your body should be in when you exercise:

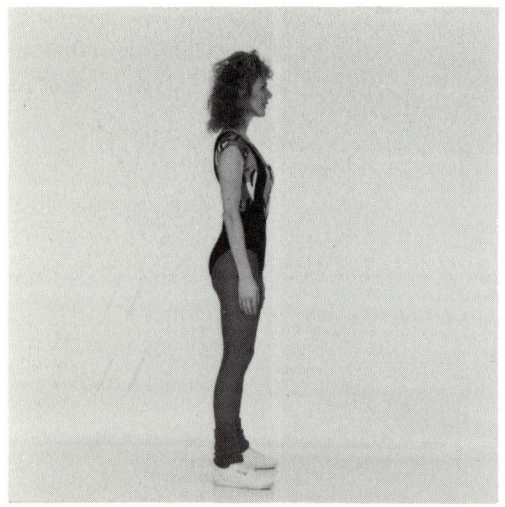

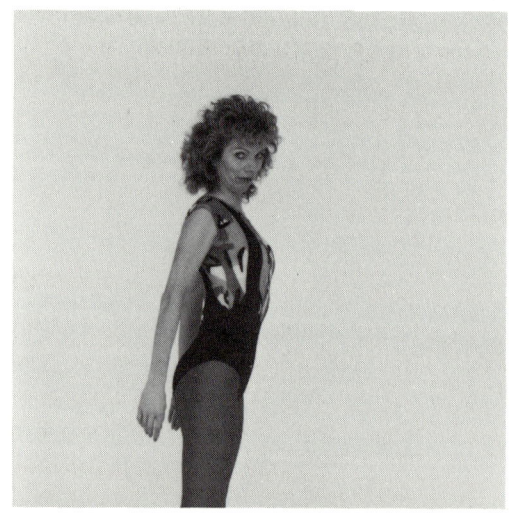

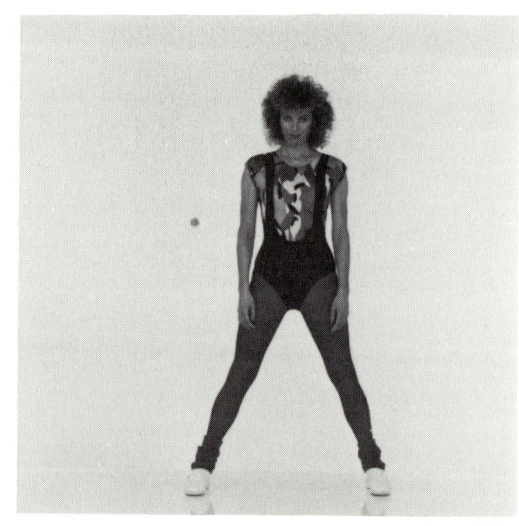

1 Check your posture. Your head should be poised, eyes looking straight in front, neck muscles relaxed, shoulders down. Your arms should hang loosely by your sides.

2 *Don't* stick out your bottom, this causes an exaggerated curve of the spine. Tuck your bottom under and pull in your tummy. Relax your knees.

3 *Don't* stand with your legs and feet too wide apart. In this illustration the gap is too big for the right body balance. Find your comfortable distance.

THE DOS AND DON'TS OF EXERCISE

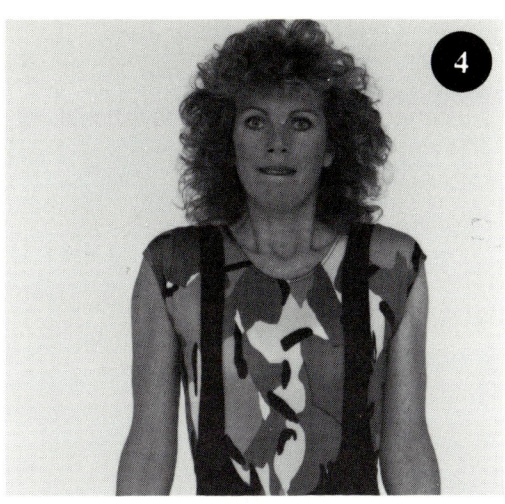

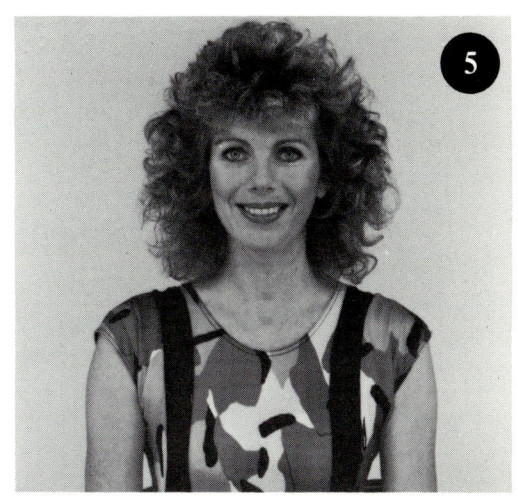

4 Concentration and effort can cause tension in the shoulders and strain the neck. Over the years, I've seen many a fervent exerciser bite their bottom lip.

5 Relax those facial muscles, enjoy the freedom of movement filling your space – smile!

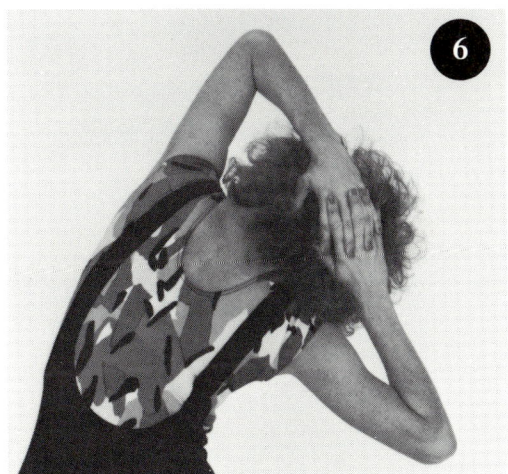

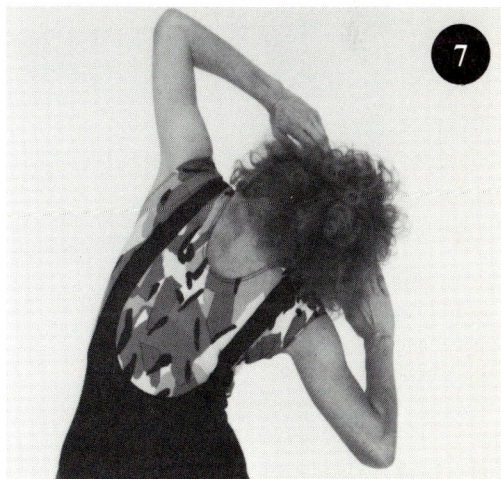

6 To avoid putting undue load on the neck muscles, when you exercise the waist and raise your arms, do not hold your hands behind your head. With the effort of the exercise this can cause too much pressure on the back of your head and neck.

7 Instead, place them on the *side* of your head with your fingertips lightly touching. This also applies to tummy exercises on the floor.

THE DOS AND DON'TS OF EXERCISE

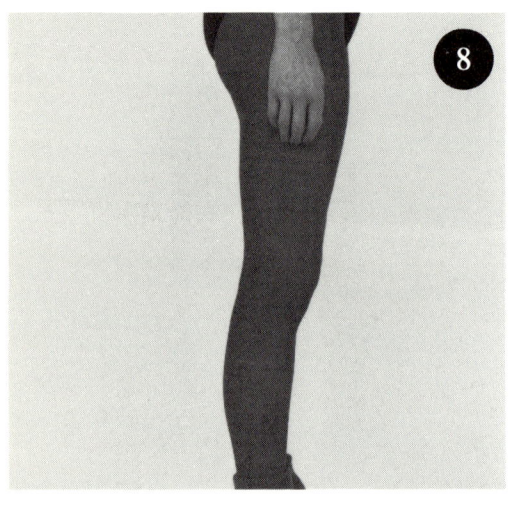

8 Kneecaps should not be pushed into the back of the knees — and the muscles should not be rigid. This is difficult to 'unlearn' if you have had ballet training.

9 Knees should be 'soft' and relaxed and only slightly tucked up on to the kneecaps.

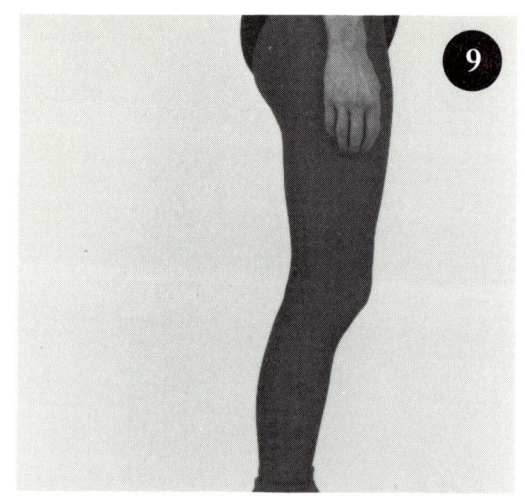

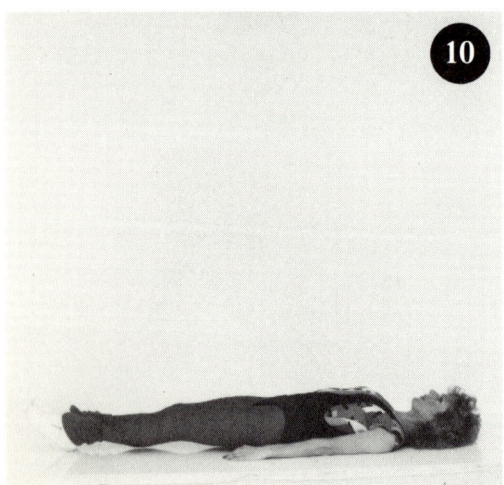

10 When lying down the small of the back should be pressed to the floor. Arching the back can weaken the spine and lead to injury.

11 Instead, draw the knees up so that the curve of the spine relaxes into the floor. This is particularly important whilst working on the tummy exercises.

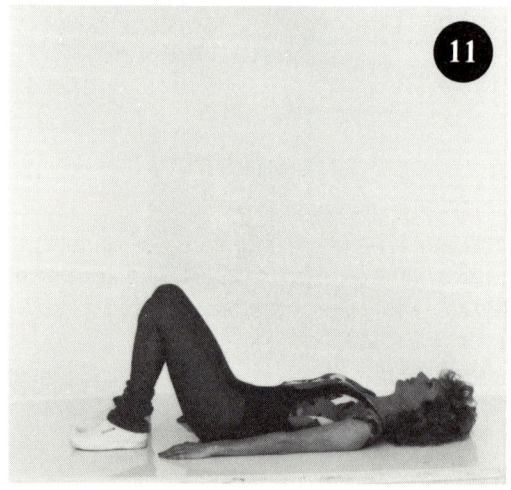

THE DOS AND DON'TS OF EXERCISE

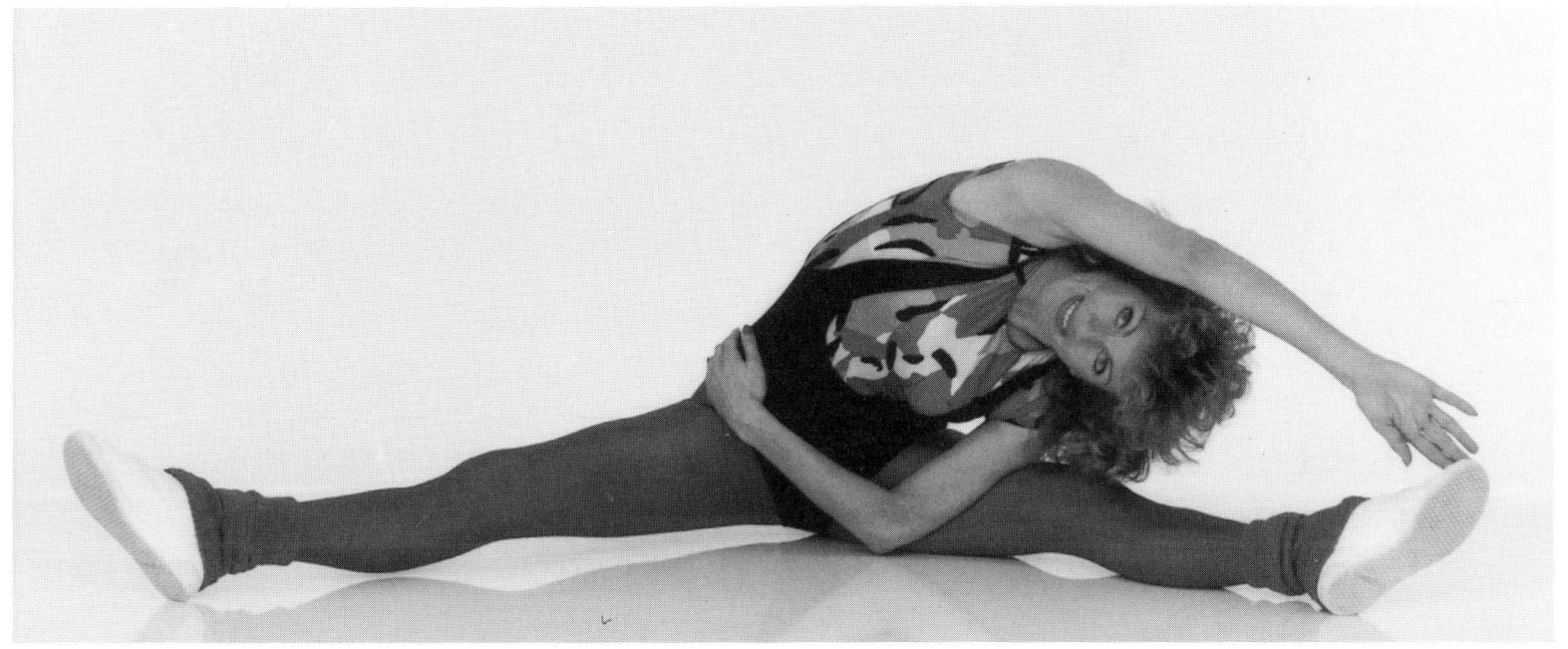

12 The temptation to overstretch whilst exercising is too great: you'll want results quickly and you might still be under the impression that to be in pain after an exercise session implies that you have worked hard. It doesn't and you shouldn't.

How Fit are You?

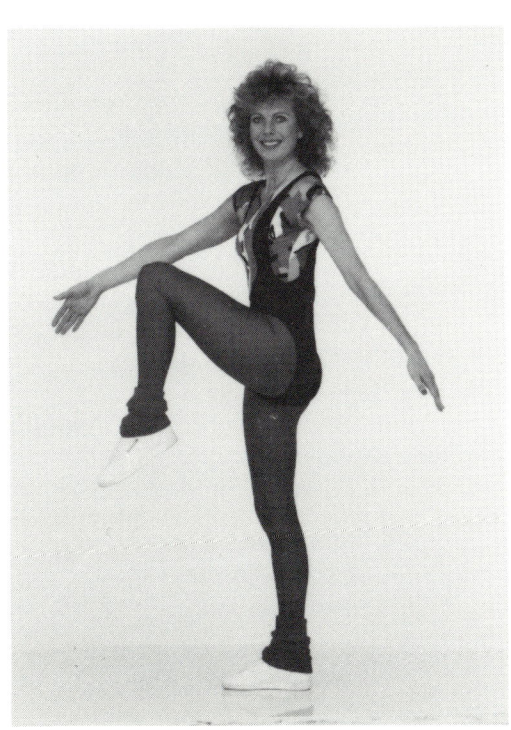

The great motivation behind regular exercise is that, done the right way, you are doing nothing but good for yourself — you are investing in a better, healthier body.

You can monitor your own progress with these tests. The three 'Ss' — Strength, Stamina and Suppleness — are what you should be aiming for, and they can all be achieved by using the workouts in this book. Your fitness goal is to ensure that, in your everyday life, no task is going to leave you breathless, your body will not be strained by lifting heavy objects and sudden movement or constant bending down will not be impeded by stiffening joints and torn muscles. These workouts will not turn you into an Olympic athlete or a star dancer, but — who knows? — they could spur you on to greater heights!

Always do a warm-up before attempting any of these tests. Keep to the sequence of tests as illustrated here, and test yourself once a week. The progress charts on pages 17 and 133 should be filled in monthly — that way you can really see the benefits of regular exercise. Make sure your muscles are warm and relaxed and have a good 'shake-out' of your shoulders, arms and legs before you begin.

HOW FIT ARE YOU?

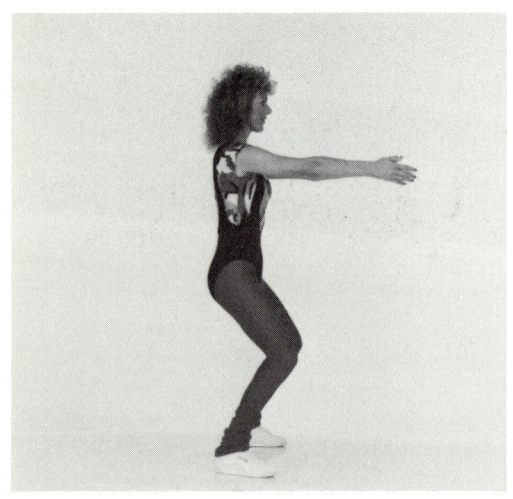 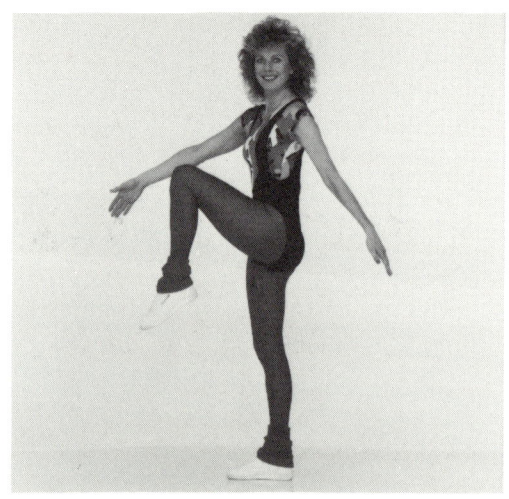 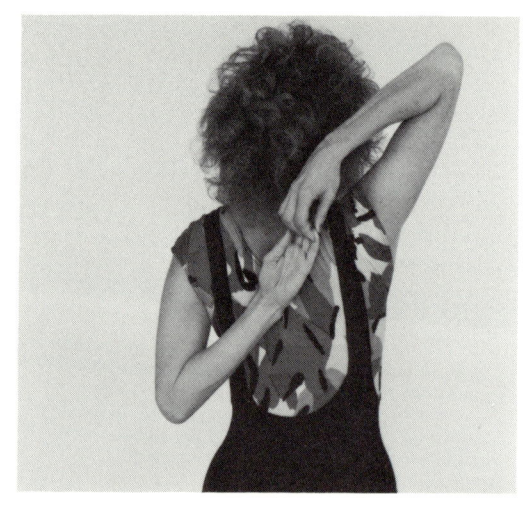

THIGH HOLD
Stand with your feet and legs a comfortable distance apart, toes facing front, arms outstretched in front, directly in line with your legs. Bend your legs, keeping your feet flat on the floor. How long can you hold this position? Straighten up and relax as soon as your thighs feel any strain, and shake out the legs. Now repeat this test, this time with your toes pointed out a little. ULTIMATE ACHIEVEMENT: ONE MINUTE

HIGH MARCHING
Raising each leg as high as possible, march on the spot. Swing your arms as you do when walking — the opposite arm to the raised leg. Control your foot as it comes down, don't crash it down on the floor, lightly place and work through the foot to raise each leg. ULTIMATE ACHIEVEMENT: 80–100 PACES

SHOULDER SUPPLENESS
Bend your left arm behind your back. Raise your right arm, bend it at the elbow and attempt to clasp your fingertips together behind your back. Now try this exercise with the other side — you will probably find that you have one shoulder that is more flexible than the other. ULTIMATE ACHIEVEMENT: CLASPING FINGERTIPS OF BOTH HANDS BEHIND YOUR BACK ON EITHER SIDE

HOW FIT ARE YOU?

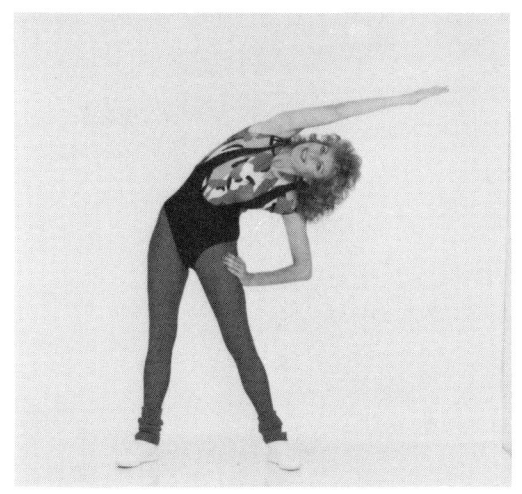 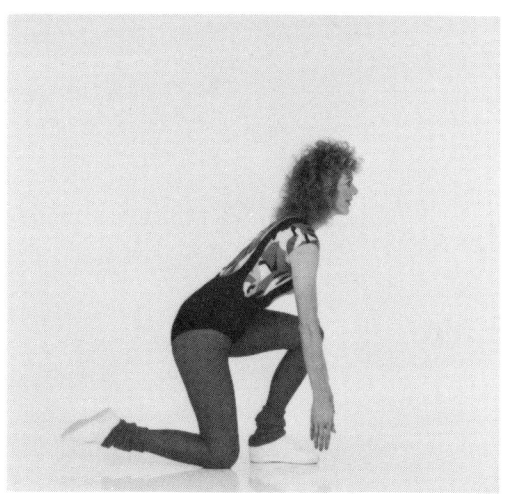 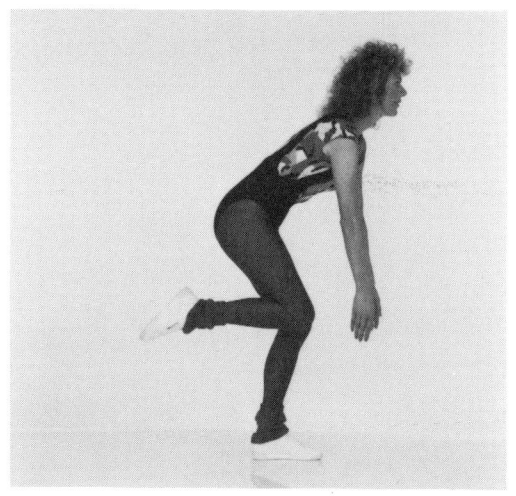

TORSO STRETCH
With your feet and legs a comfortable distance apart, raise your left arm and place your right hand on the top of your right thigh. Lean directly to your right side. Centralize and repeat, changing sides. Check your position — with *any* waist exercise you should rise out of the hips before leaning. Also, there should be no tilting backwards or forwards. ULTIMATE ACHIEVEMENT: REACHING OVER TO A NINETY DEGREE ANGLE ON BOTH SIDES

ULTIMATE THIGH TEST
Kneel on your right knee, lean forward and upright. Raise the toes of your right foot off the ground. →

Keeping your left foot flat on the floor, and *without* your right foot touching the ground, stand up. Some people — including several sports personalities — have tried this test with me on television, and never managed it! It helps to lean forward, and swinging the arms behind and then forward as you stand up gives you added impetus. Try the other leg. You will find a definite difference in strength between your left and right thighs. ULTIMATE ACHIEVEMENT: TO STAND UP WITH EASE, WITHOUT LEANING FORWARD, ON *BOTH* LEGS

HOW FIT ARE YOU?

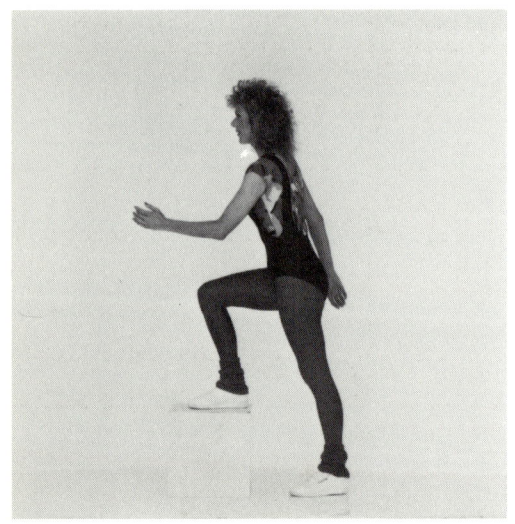

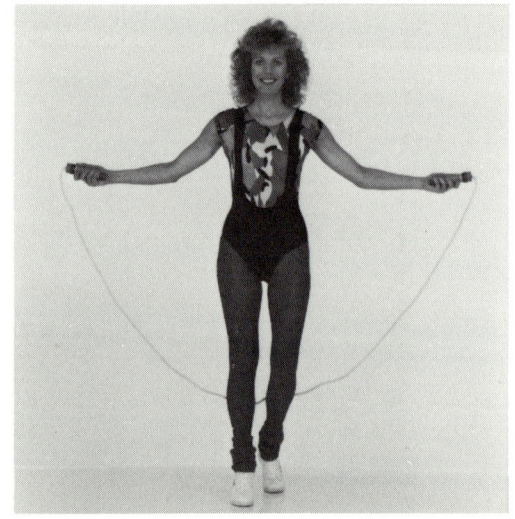

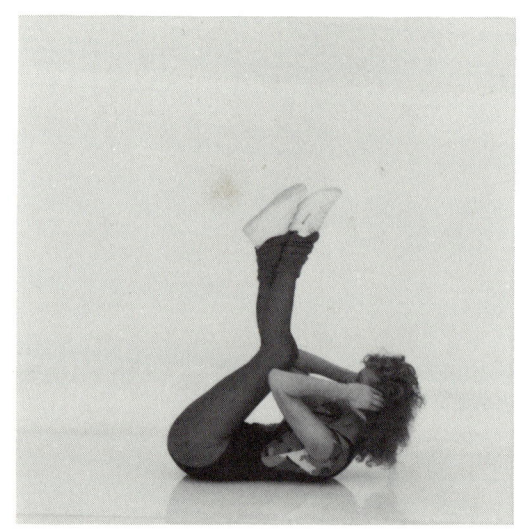

STAMINA
Using a steep stair or solid box, step up with your right, then your left foot, and down right, down left. Keep it rhythmical and as you get fitter increase the pace. ULTIMATE ACHIEVEMENT: TO CONTINUE THIS TEST FOR ONE FULL MINUTE AND AIM TO EXTEND THE LENGTH OF TIME EACH TIME YOU TEST YOURSELF

AEROBIC
With a skipping rope, lightly skip at a fast pace. Your skipping will improve with practice. You can keep yourself entertained by crossing your skipping rope and changing footwork. ULTIMATE ACHIEVEMENT: TO SKIP FOR 4–5 MINUTES – AND WANT TO DO MORE!

TUMMY STRENGTH
Lying on your back, lightly place your hands at the side of your head and cross your legs in the air at the ankles. Keep your head off the ground at all times. In a small rocking motion, reach forward, elbows touching knees (or beyond) and back. Exhale as you touch your knees. ULTIMATE ACHIEVEMENT: 50+

Progress Chart

Test yourself every month and complete this chart.

THIGH HOLD
Time yourself. How long can you comfortably hold this exercise?
a) feet in b) feet out

HIGH MARCHING
How many can you do?

SHOULDER SUPPLENESS
Fill in when your fingertips are:
a) nearly touching b) touching c) firmly grasping – both sides

TORSO STRETCH

ULTIMATE THIGH TEST
Fill in when you can rise up:
a) with difficulty b) to a standing position
c) without leaning forward

STAMINA
How long can you continuously step up and down?

AEROBIC
How long can you skip? Either count or time yourself

TUMMY
How many can you do?

JAN	FEB	MAR	APR	MAY	JUN

Monday

WARM UP Try each exercise eight times, but only attempt the amount you are capable of — this might only be four of each exercise to begin with.

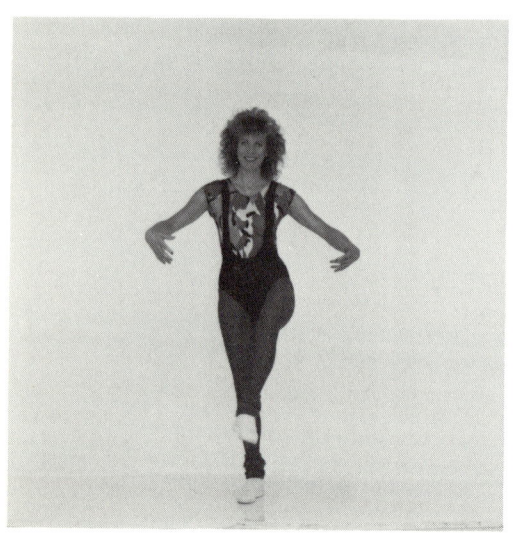 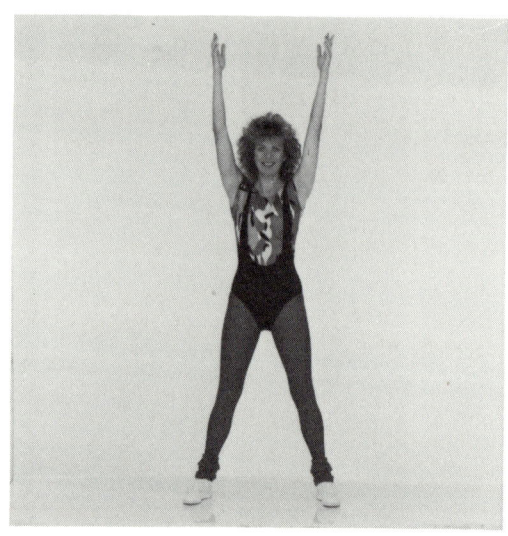 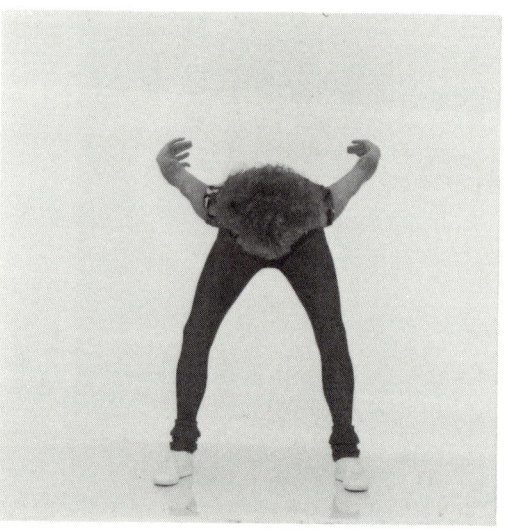

'Shake out' to relax the muscles, loosely shake out the arms, hands and shoulders, followed by the legs and feet.

Stand tall, feet and legs apart, arms raised above your head. →

Bend your legs, as in skiing. As you do so, swing your arms down and behind. Now swing back and straighten up.

MONDAY: WARM UP

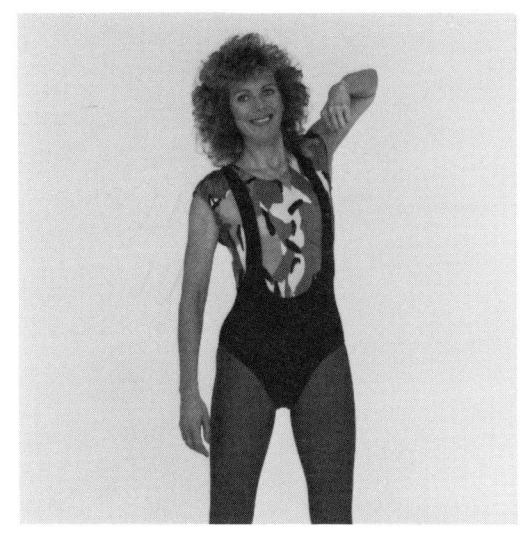 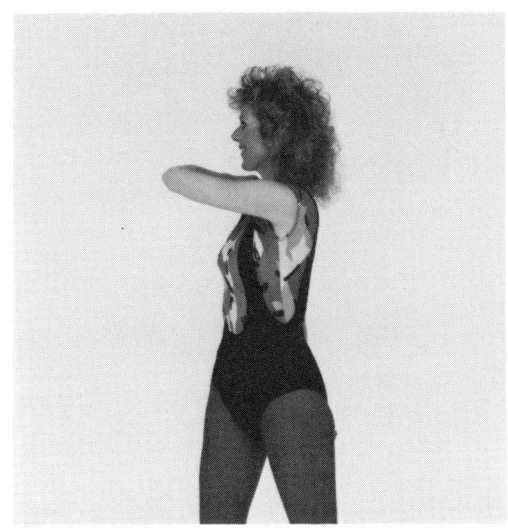 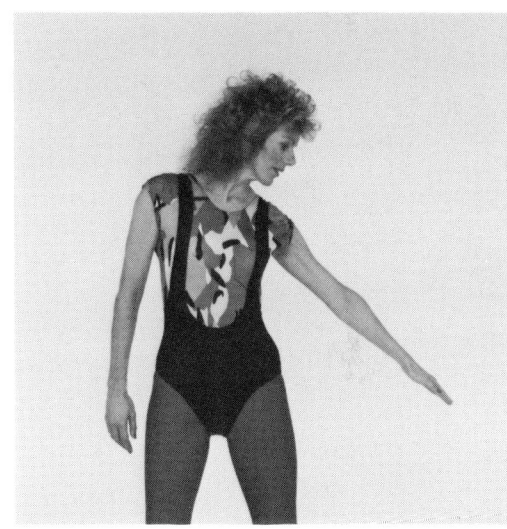

Bend your right arm and, guided by your elbow, circle your shoulder. Complete eight circles and repeat with your left arm.

Bend your right arm across your body at shoulder height and, as you do so, turn from your waist to look to your left. →

Swing your arm back down diagonally across your body. Continue flowing these two movements together, and repeat with your left arm.

MONDAY: WARM UP

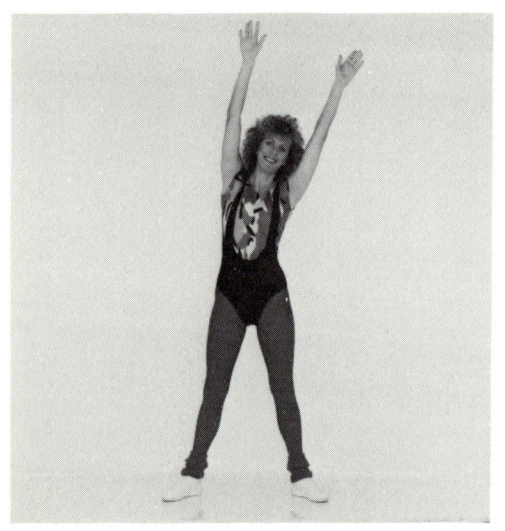 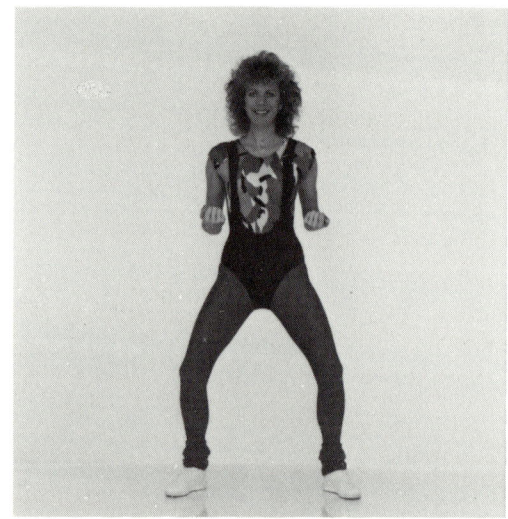 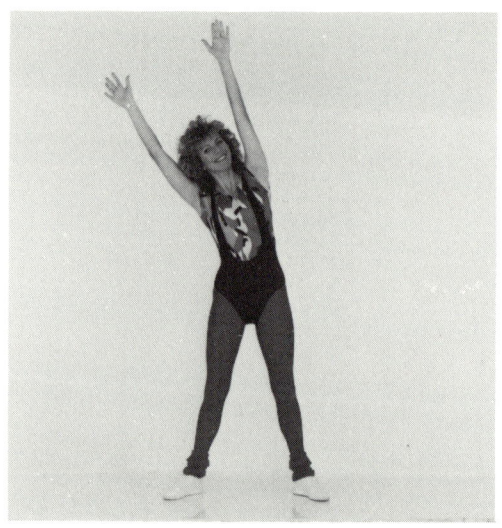

Raise both your arms up to your right diagonal. Stretch up out of your hips, tummy in, and reach just a little more to your right. →

Bend your legs as you bring both arms in, elbows tucked into the sides of the body. →

And stretch up with both arms, reaching for your left diagonal. Bend your legs again, drawing in both arms to your sides and keep flowing this exercise through these three movements.

MONDAY: WARM UP

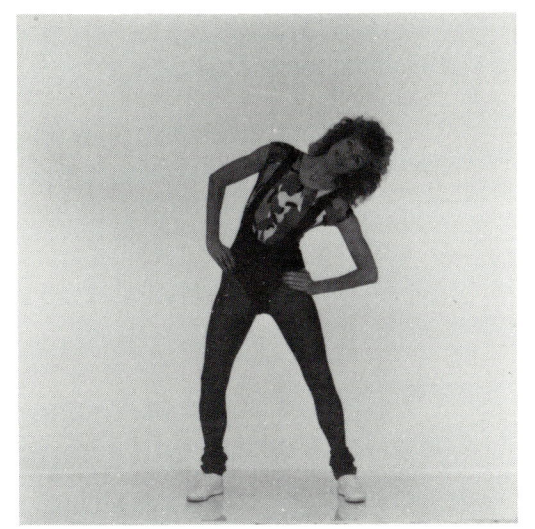

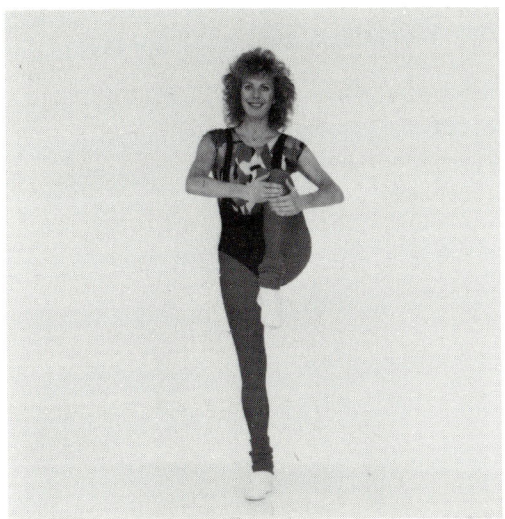

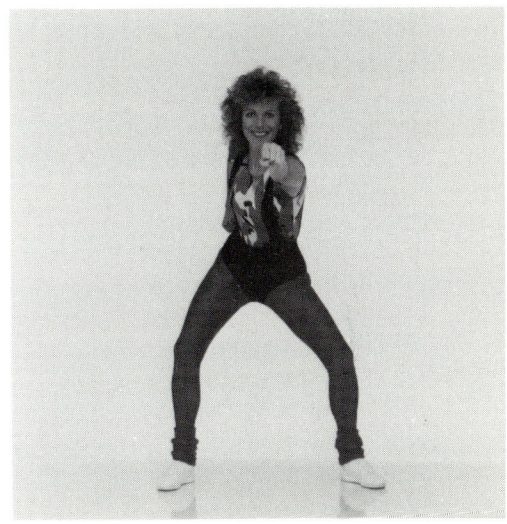

Bend your legs a little, place your hands at the top of your thighs and lean directly to your right side. Slowly centralize, and repeat the lean to your left side. Continue slowly stretching and working the waist in this way.

Raise your right knee and, lightly clasping it just below the knee with both hands, ease your leg up, helping to loosen both the leg and your right hip. Repeat the exercise with your left leg.

To complete your warm-up, think of all the things you would really like to hit — and punch through the air instead! Bend your legs and alternate punching out in front with each arm, using the strength of the shoulders. Hit hard, through to the fists.

Then 'shake out' as you did at the beginning!

MONDAY: WAIST

WAIST

After the weekend, Monday is definitely the day to tone up and trim the waistline. Do as many of these exercises as you can. You might prefer to select the first four and keep practising them before you attempt the harder ones. See how many you can do, and gradually increase the number you can achieve of each exercise.

The amount of reaching and stretching should be minimal: the movements should be tiny and repetitious.

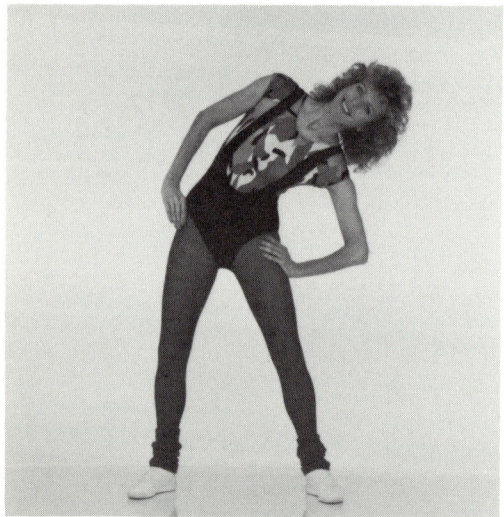

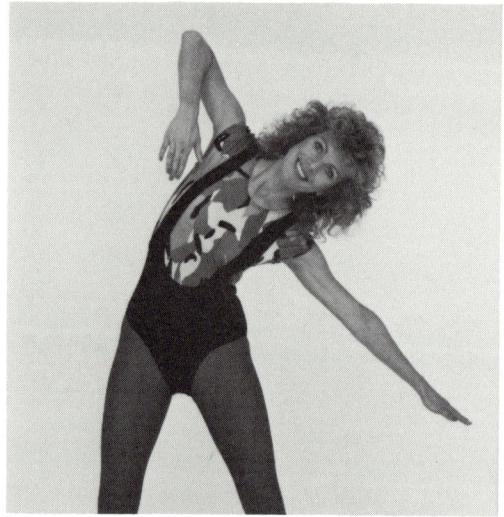

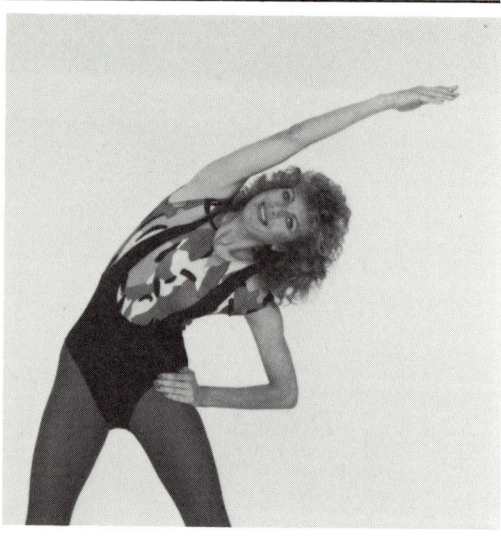

Place your hands at the top of your thighs and lean to your right. Centralize, and lean to your left.

As if cutting through the air, pull your left elbow up as your right arm reaches down and out. Straighten up, bringing both elbows together in front and repeat to the left.

Place your right hand at the top of your thigh and reach up and over with your left. Reach over with a tiny, stretching movement. Change sides.

MONDAY: WAIST

Keep the kneecaps relaxed, your feet and legs a comfortable distance apart. There should be no twisting—you should lean only to your side—and no tilting of the torso, forwards or backwards.

The secret of a firm, shapely waistline is regular waist exercise.

Always think 'pull up to go over' before any waist exercise — it will help you to get used to rising out of your hips before stretching to the side — that is the correct way to exercise the waist.

Your aim is to achieve eight of each exercise on both sides of the body.

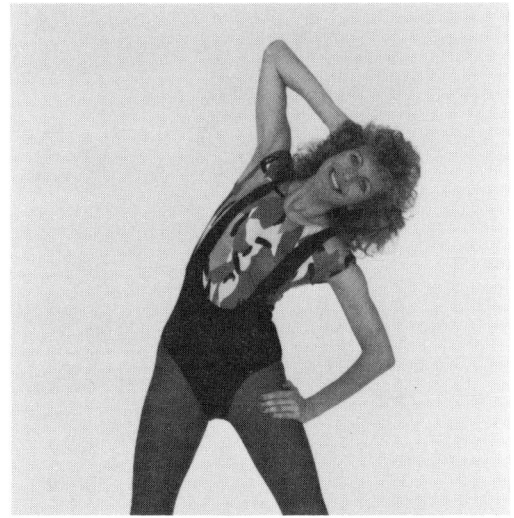

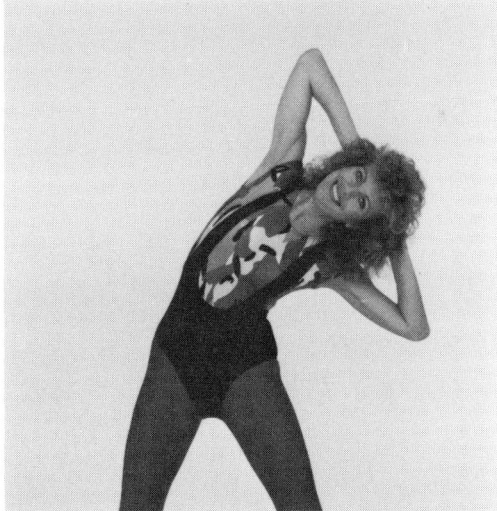

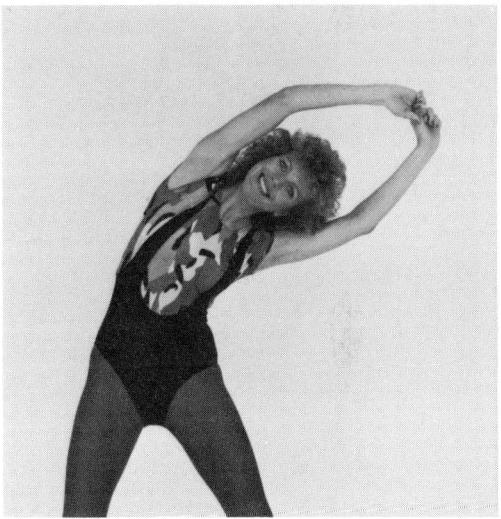

Stand straight, place your left hand at the side of your head and your right hand at the top of your right thigh. Repeat the lean of the previous exercise to the right and the left.

This time, exercise the waist by copying the previous exercise, but with both hands placed lightly at the side of your head.

Clasp your hands together over your head and reach out over to your right side. Hold your fingers together as you then stretch them straight over your head. Repeat to the left.

23

MONDAY: WAIST

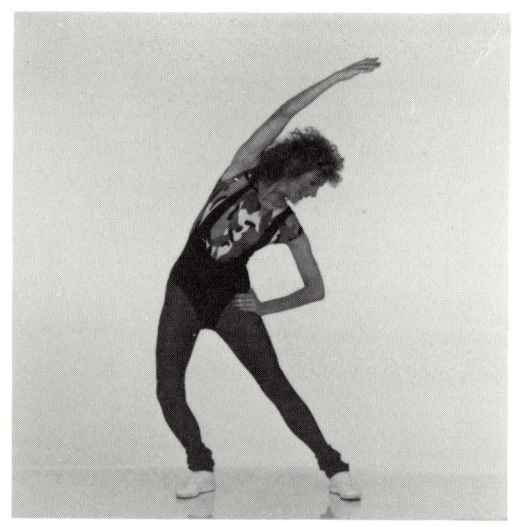 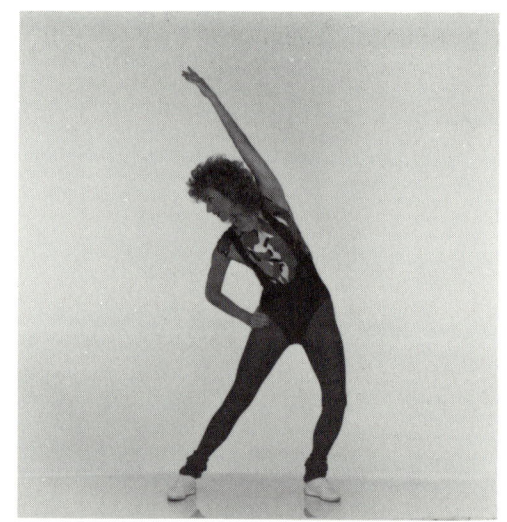 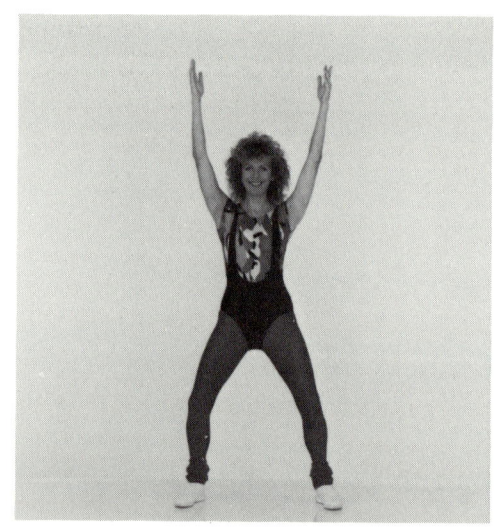

Bend your left leg and straighten the right. Arc your left arm over your head and, as you stretch over, feel the gentle pull on your left side. Gently stretch in that position with tiny movements. →

Repeat to your left, feeling the stretch right up the right side of your body.

Raise both arms above your head and bend both legs. →

MONDAY: WAIST

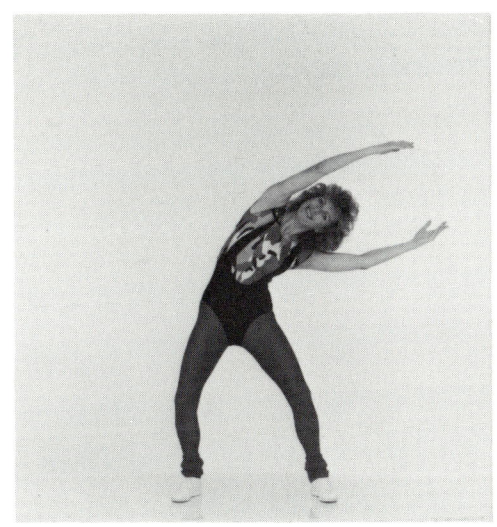

Lean to your right side. →

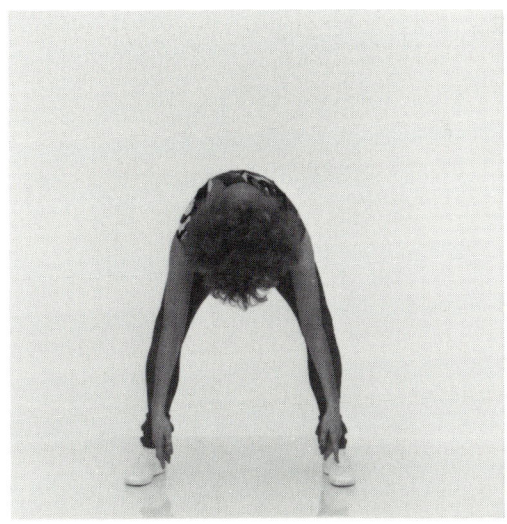

Continue round in the circle to your toes, and hang like a rag doll. →

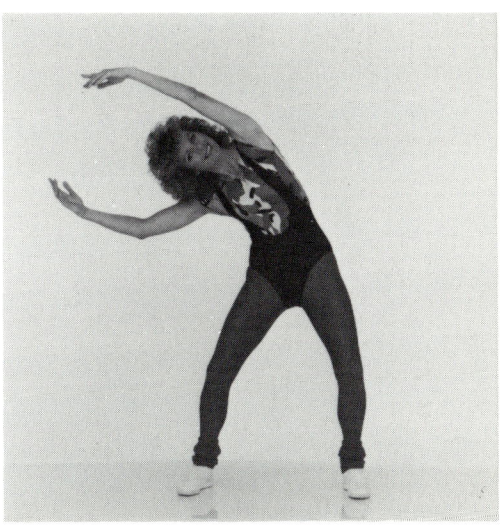

Rise up to your left side, both arms rising up with you, and finish back at the centre. Repeat and change sides.

MONDAY: TUMMY STAGE I

TUMMY STAGE I

Get to grips with these tummy exercises. This is stage one, and you might need to select just some of these exercises and concentrate on being able to do each one at least eight times before going on to the others.

If you are not used to exercising regularly it will take you longer to build up the muscle power before attempting the stage two exercises on Thursday.

Remember to work through a curved spine and to keep the movements smooth and minimal. Always breathe out with the effort of the exercise (e.g. when you are sitting up) and breathe in when you lie back.

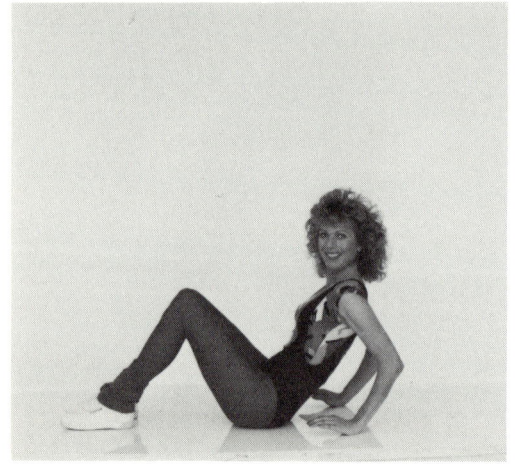
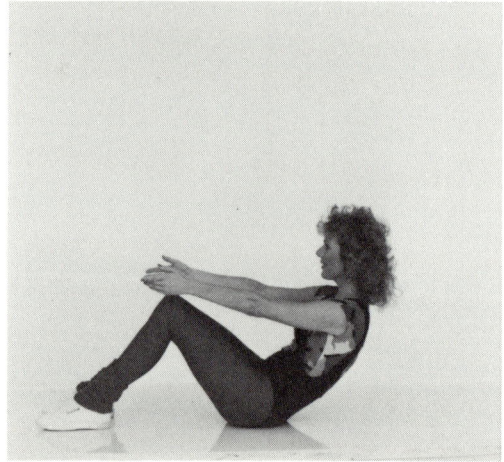
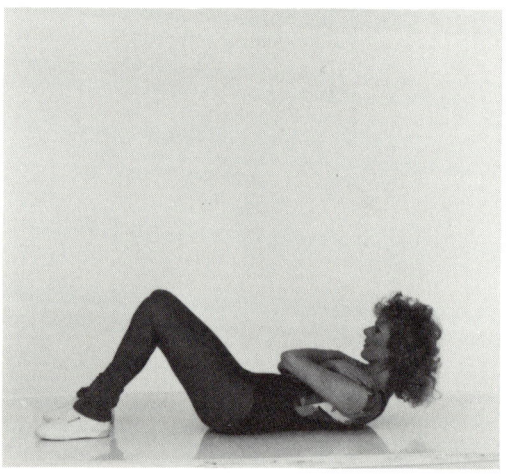

Sit on the floor with feet and legs a small distance apart, legs drawn up, feet flat on the floor. Place your hands at either side of your body — to give extra support to those slack tummy muscles. Lean back and then forwards in a rocking motion, pushing through the hands if necessary.

After a while you will be able to do the previous exercise without the aid of your hands. With both arms in front, sink back, hold that position and slowly sit up again. Repeat.

Lie on the floor, legs drawn up, feet flat. With your arms crossed over your chest, raise your head off the floor. On beat two, sit up a little more, and on three even more. Lie back slowly in three stages, relax and repeat. See how many you can do.

MONDAY: TUMMY STAGE I

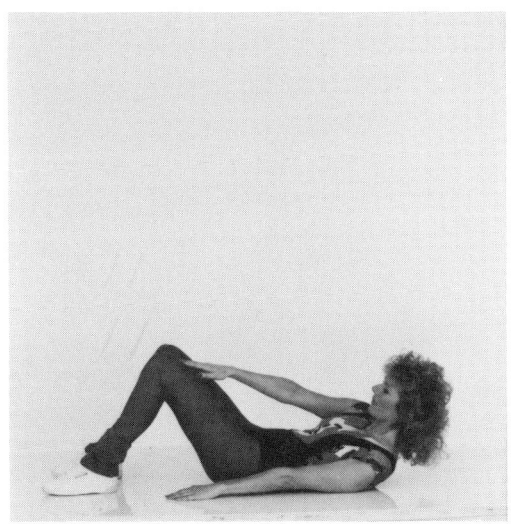 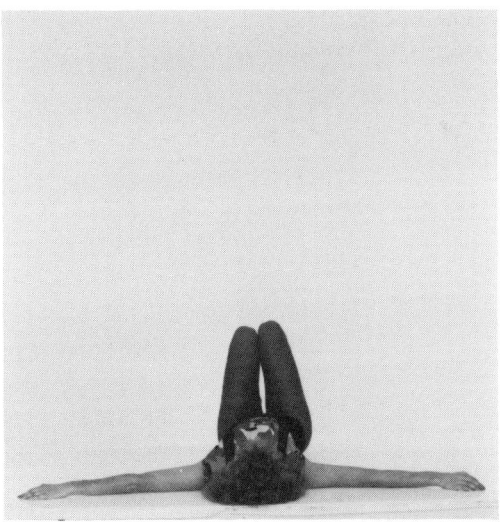 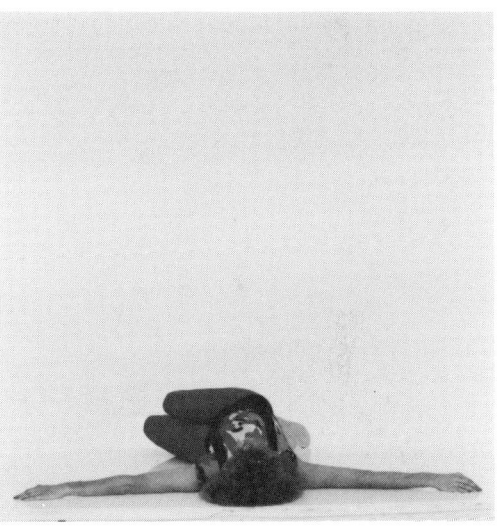

This time the head stays off the floor for the entire exercise. This is a quick repetitious exercise. Reach for your left knee with your right fingers, sitting up off your shoulders. Lie back (but not on your head) and change to reach for your right knee with your left fingers.

Slow the pace down and feel your tummy flatten as you lie flat on your back with your arms outstretched to the side. Both knees are drawn up and stay together as you point your toes together on the floor. →

Working from the waist, let both knees roll over to your left side. Your knees probably won't touch the floor, and neither will your shoulders — but give it time and practice. Lift your knees back to the centre and repeat, rolling them to your right.

MONDAY: TUMMY STAGE I

For these exercises, keep your head off the floor — do not let it fall back.

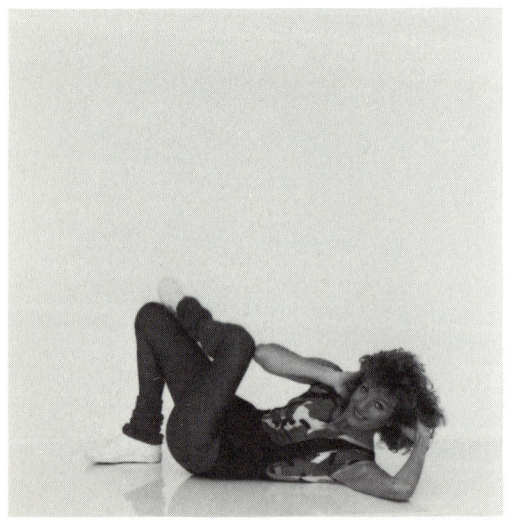 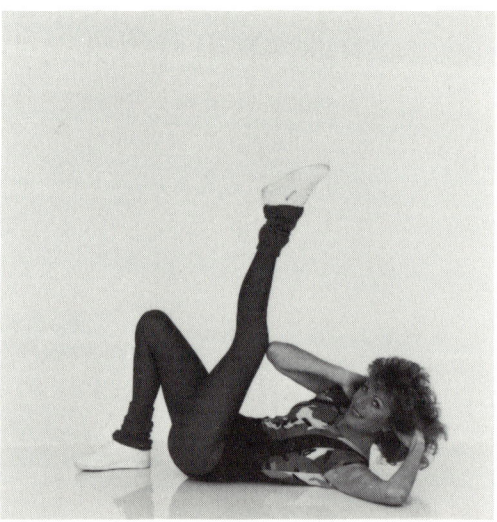 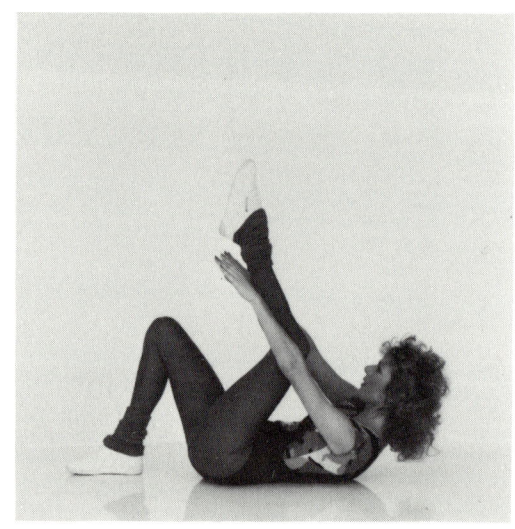

Bend your right leg, keeping the foot flat on the floor. Cross your left leg over it, resting the foot just above the right knee. In quick repetitive movements sit up and back, touching your left knee with your right elbow. Change sides and repeat.

This time extend your left leg in the air and touch your left knee with your right elbow. Lie back and repeat. Change sides.

Bend your left leg in the air, with the thigh well back. Keep 'sitting' up and back only as high as in the illustration. Change legs.

MONDAY: TUMMY STAGE I

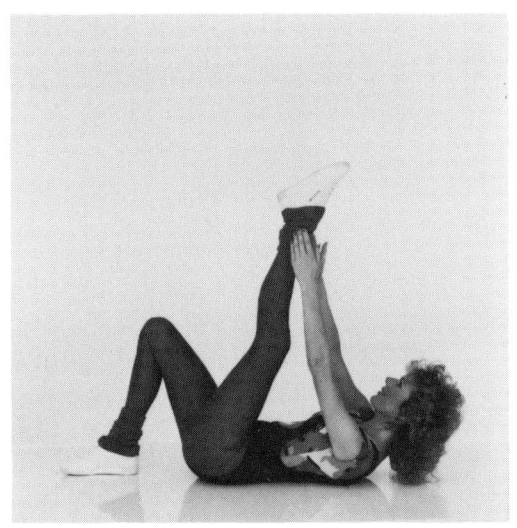 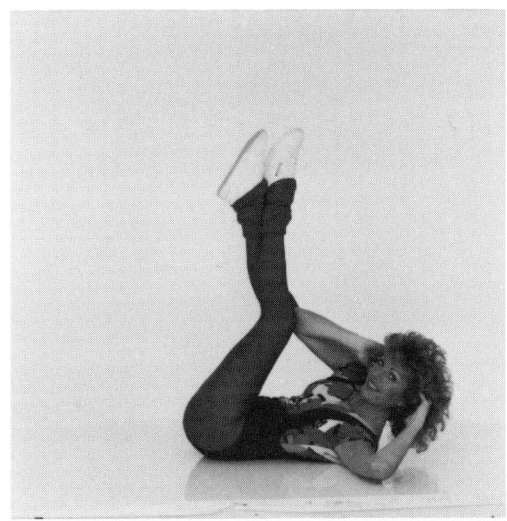 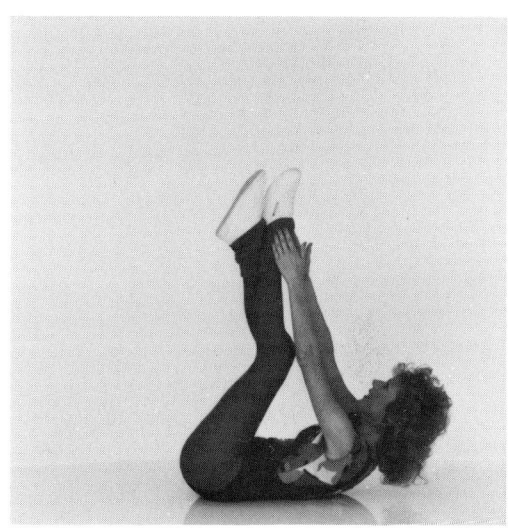

Extend your left leg in the air and reach up with your hands, arms stretched up. Lie back only as far as the shoulders and keep reaching up and back in a small, rhythmical movement.

Cross your legs in the air, locking them at the ankles. Sit up to touch your knees with your right elbow, working across the body. Lie back on the shoulders (not the head) and take your left elbow across the body to touch the knees. This is a fast, continuous exercise.

Finally, still with your feet locked in the air, reach up and back for your ankles.

MONDAY: HIPS, THIGHS AND BOTTOM STAGE I

HIPS, THIGHS AND BOTTOM STAGE I

Oh that troublesome area! Women collect fat in these three areas — men in the tummy (that's why we see so many unfit 'pregnant' men around!). There are more fat cells in a woman's body, and there are three main stages in a woman's life when the hips, thighs and bottom might be prone to accumulating fat: adolescence, pregnancy and menopause — all times of great hormonal

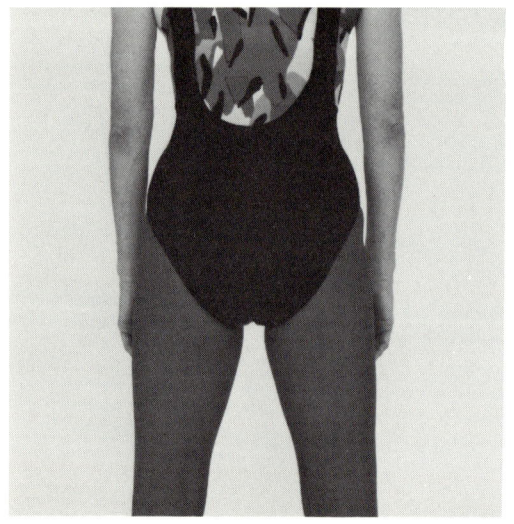 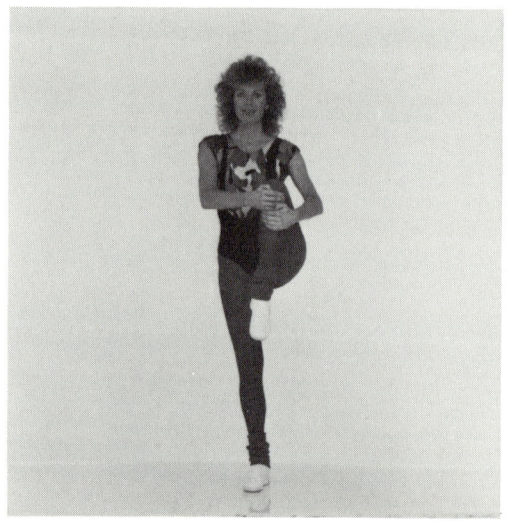 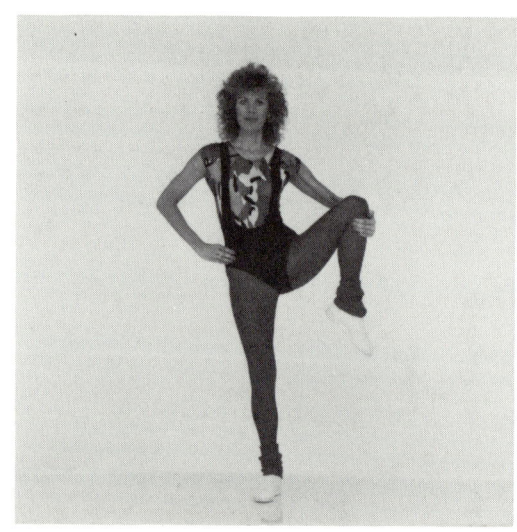

You can do this exercise sitting down, standing at a bus stop or at the kitchen sink — and nobody is going to know. Clench and relax your buttocks — eight times with your right, eight with your left, and as many as you can with both.

Stand straight. Raise your right knee, hold it just below the knee with both hands and lower the leg. Keep repeating before changing legs.

Repeat the same exercise, but turn the leg out to the side (this is not so easy and requires greater control and balance). Repeat and change sides.

MONDAY: HIPS, THIGHS AND BOTTOM STAGE I

change. Of course if you lead a sedentary life, exercise rarely and eat unhealthily, the problem will be exacerbated.

These exercises will help stimulate the circulation and firm up those stubborn areas.

They are easy and very effective — so take heart, there is hope for you yet! Aim to do sixteen of each exercise.

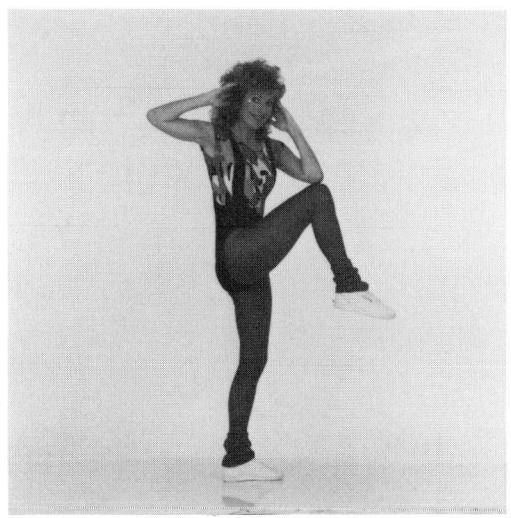

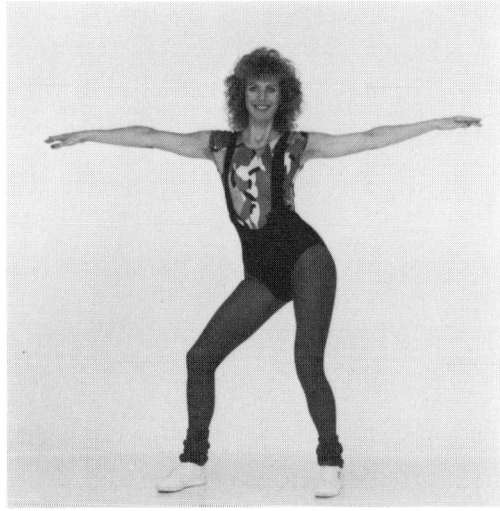

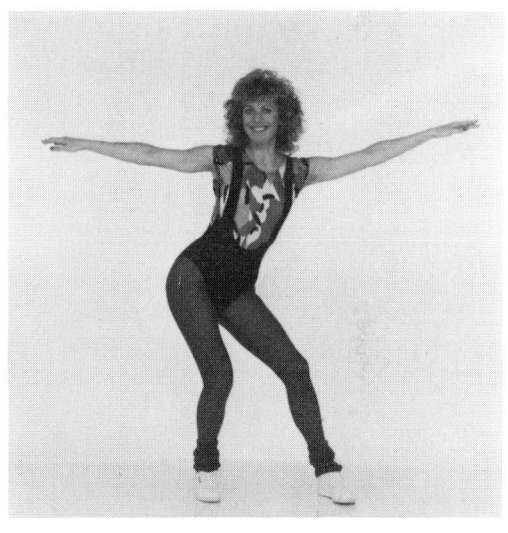

Lightly place your hands at each side of your head. Alternate raising each leg and turning to touch its knee with the opposite elbow. You will see quick results with this exercise, but try not to lean forward. If necessary, bend both legs at the same time.

Think of a circle and circle your trunk. Keeping both legs bent, guide your hips round to the right and continue to the front. →

Circle round to the left and then behind, making continuous circles.

MONDAY: HIPS, THIGHS AND BOTTOM STAGE I

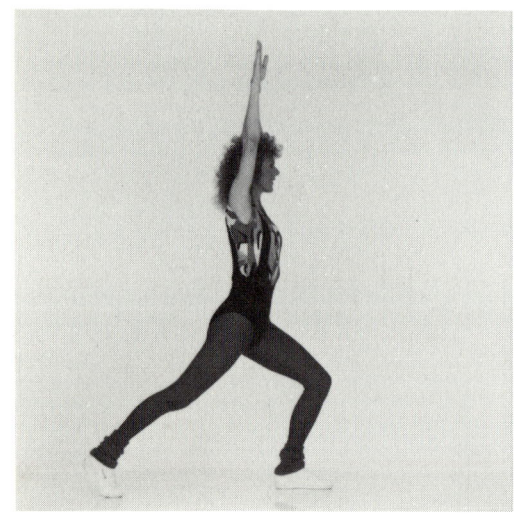 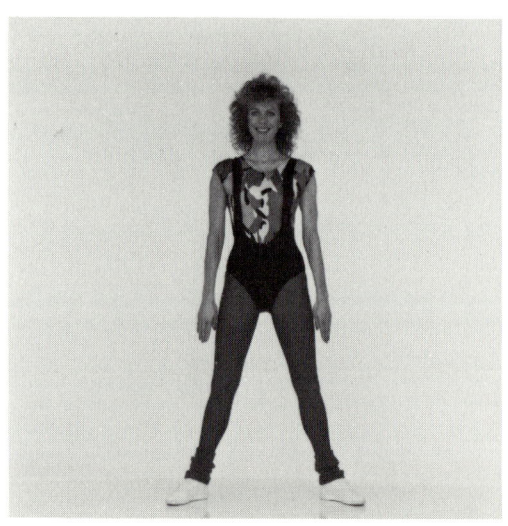 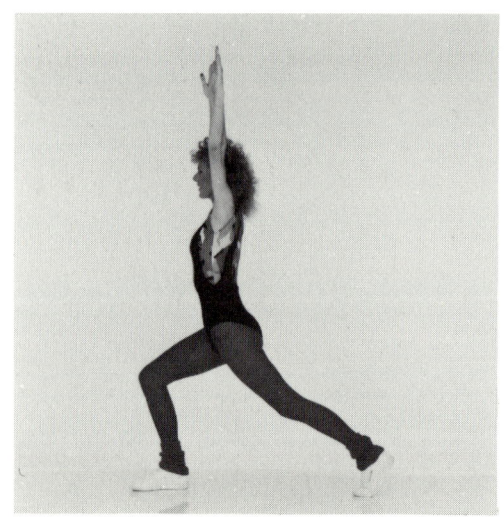

Facing your right side, lunge forward and step on a bent right leg. Raise both arms simultaneously forward and up. →

Straighten up facing the front and lowering the arms. →

On the next count, step forward on your left leg facing your left side. Repeat.

MONDAY: HIPS, THIGHS AND BOTTOM STAGE I

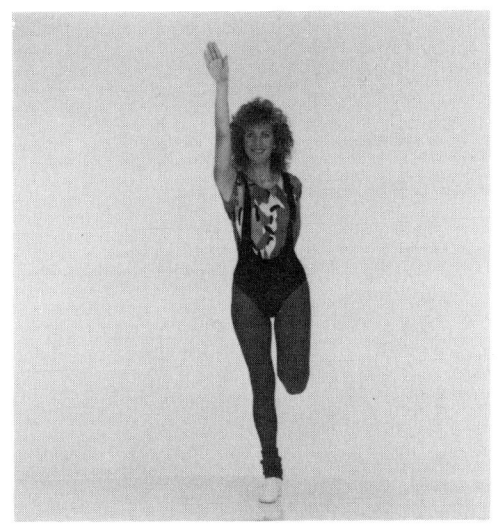
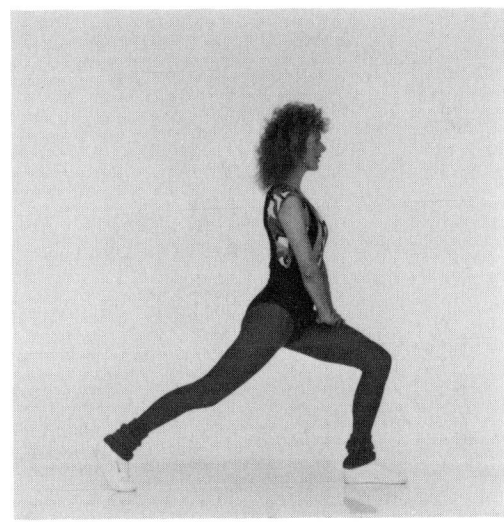
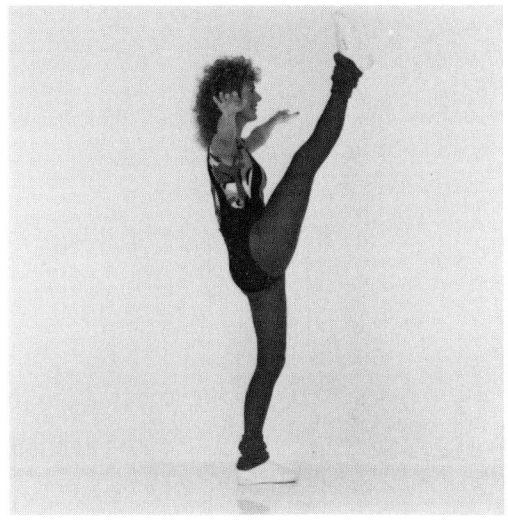

Balance on your left leg, raise your left arm and bend your right leg so that your right knee is tucked in close to your left leg. Hold on to your right foot with your right hand. Feel the stretch on the thigh and hold that position for approximately 30 seconds. Change legs (but do not repeat).

Bend your left leg in front of you with your right leg stretched out behind. →

Kick your right leg straight up in front, arms stretched for balance. Don't over kick — you might only kick to waist height — place your leg behind again and repeat before changing sides.

Shake out those leg muscles!

Tuesday

WARM UP

Attempt each exercise eight times, but you must work within your physical capabilities. If you can only achieve six of each to begin with don't worry, you will soon feel able to do more!

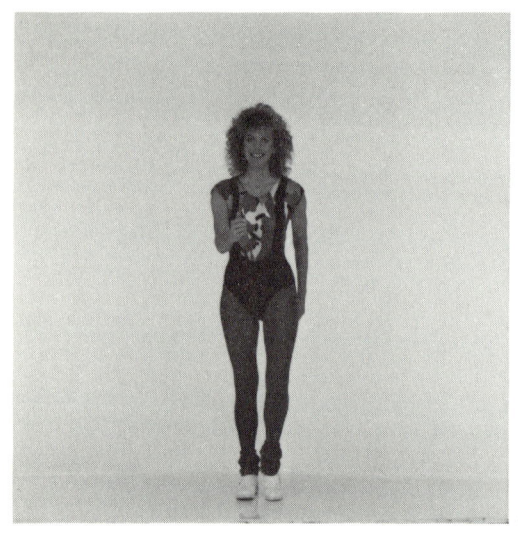 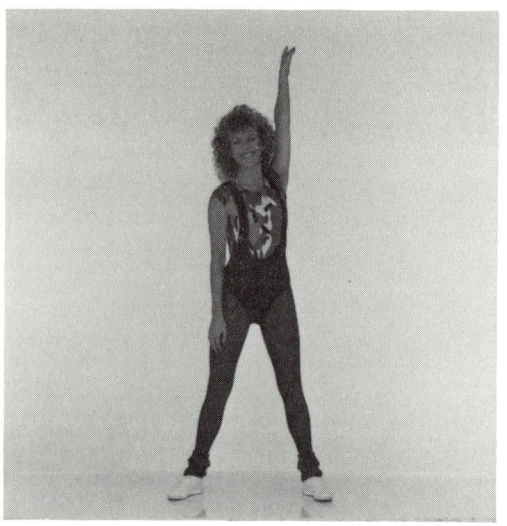 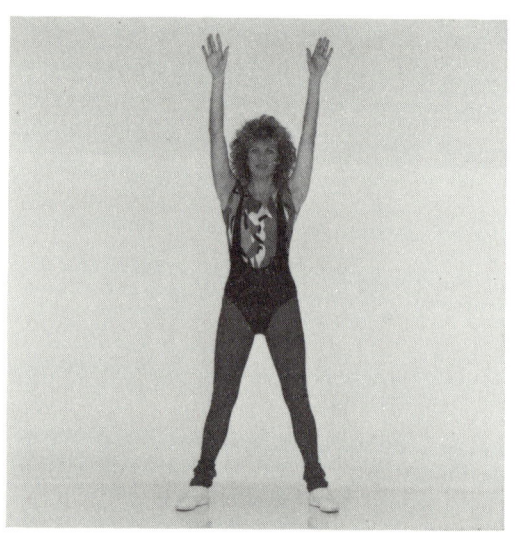

Lightly mark time on the spot, pushing through each foot and swinging each arm as if you were jogging — but without the running. Do this for about a minute.

With your feet and legs apart, circle your right arm forward and round, keeping your arm relaxed. Complete the circle eight times and repeat with your left arm.

Circle both arms together quite briskly. Feel your shoulders easing as you do so, but don't force your arms right behind you.

TUESDAY: WARM UP

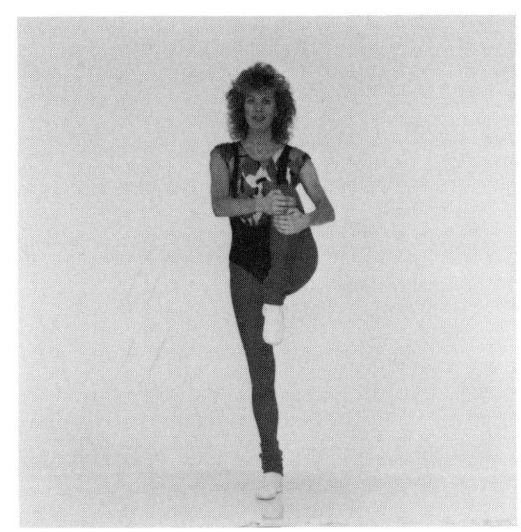 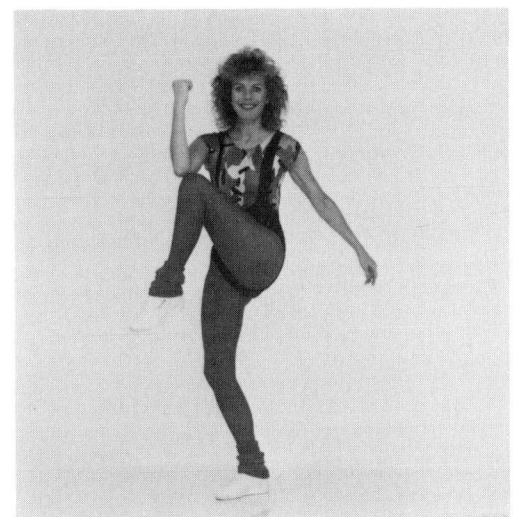 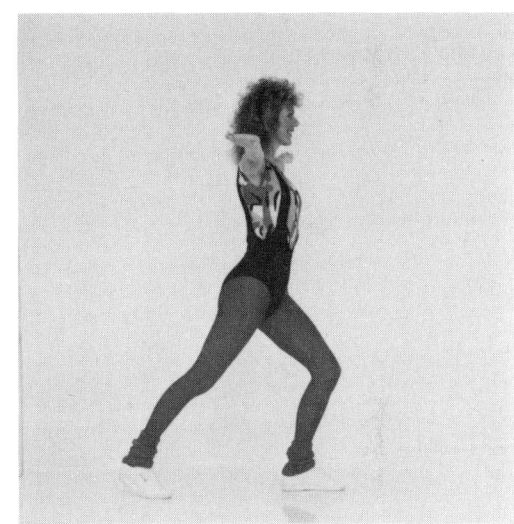

Stand straight. Raise your right knee, holding it just below the knee with both hands, and lower the leg. Repeat and change sides.

Raise your right leg, bending it across your body as high as you can. Swing your left elbow across your body at the same time, aiming to touch your knee. Lower your leg out to the side as you swing your elbow down to the side. Repeat and change sides.

Face your right side, arms outstretched at your sides, and stretch your left leg out behind you, bending your right knee and keeping your right foot flat on the floor. Hold that position, then repeat to your left.

TUESDAY: WARM UP

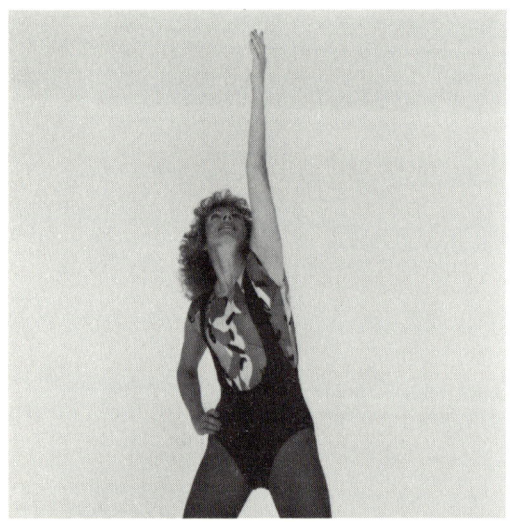

The following six movements are a sequence — each flowing into the next — to stretch your torso, trim your waist and help strengthen the back muscles. Place your left hand on your left hip and bend your legs. Reach up with your right arm and look up. →

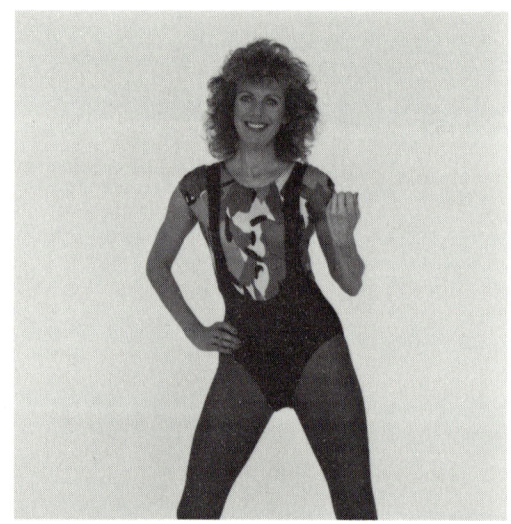

Bend your right arm into your body, making a fist. →

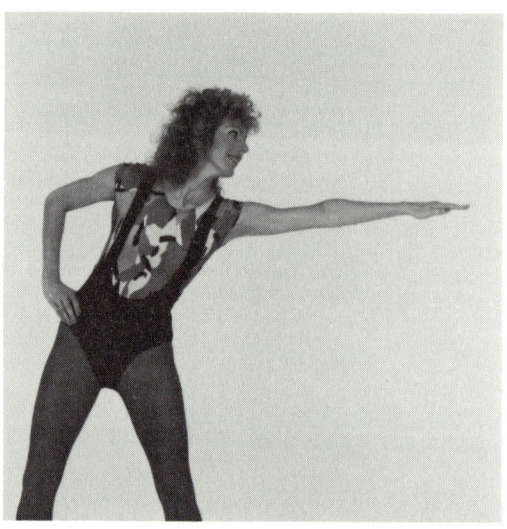

Now reach out to your right side, leaning from your hips. →

TUESDAY: WARM UP

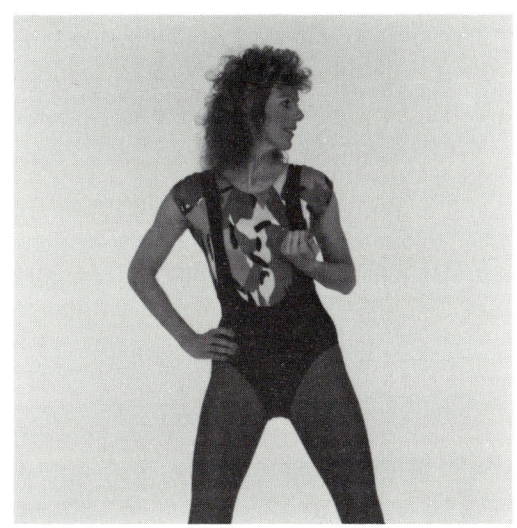

Bend your arm back into the side of your body, making a fist. →

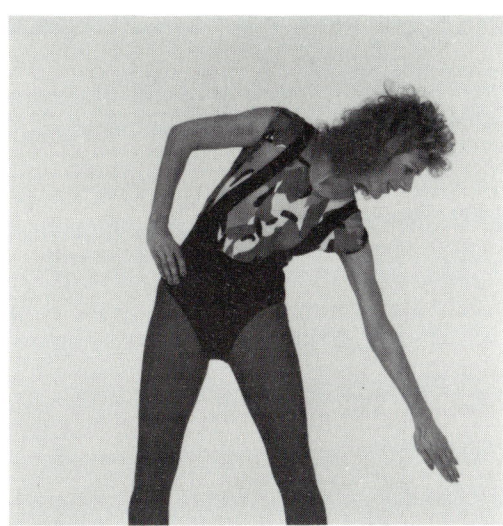

Reach down, leaning over and looking down at your fingertips. →

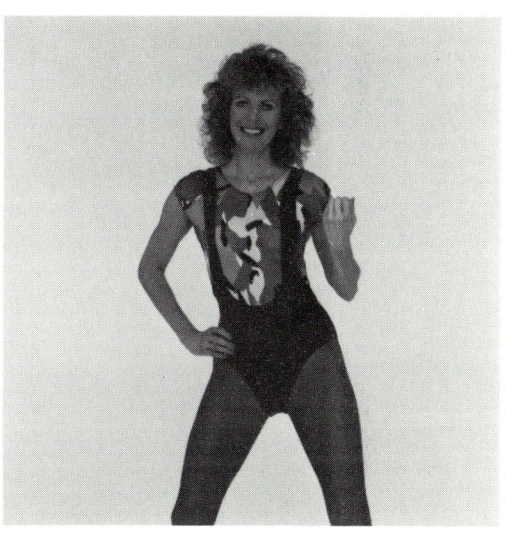

Come up again, fist drawn in, and repeat the sequence. Change to your left.

Postural Problems

Nearly all of us, at one time or another, have experienced back pain. Keeping fit helps maintain our structure, oiling and lubricating the joints, shaping and building up muscle power. Central to that body structure is the back, with all its complexities and intricacies, strengths and weaknesses. Injury to the back, however small, is likely to have the most debilitating effect on our everyday lives. Most of us could help minimize pending back problems by taking a good look at our posture.

There are three common conditions — read them carefully; then, standing sideways to a full-length mirror, turn your head and look at the way you are standing. Have you:

A Flat Back? This looks like a slouch. The muscles in the upper back have gone rigid, the lower back gets pulled flat and the whole curve is completely lost.

A Sway Back? An exaggerated curve of the spine, with the pelvis tipping forward. This is often seen in pregnant women when the large, protruding tummy in front pulls the back into this abnormal position.

A Rounded Back? If you're desk bound or spend hours sitting leaning over a table it's almost inevitable that you'll get a 'hunched' look. The large muscle at the upper half of the back pulls the back into this abnormal position.

So readjust your body in both the sitting and standing position to the correct posture.

There should be a slight curve in the neck as your head is poised, eyes looking straight ahead, shoulders relaxed, arms hanging loosely by your sides. Your bottom should be tucked under, not pushed out, this causes a strain on the smallest, weakest part of the spine. The knees should be 'tucked up' on the kneecaps, not pushed right in to the knees, and the feet should be spread a comfortable distance apart.

Deep breathing can also help with posture. Too often we take shallow breaths. When you take a deep breath you use the lower back muscles and this helps both the lower and upper back to sit in their correct positions, and helps the muscles either side of your spine to relax.

Deep breathing is also good for our overall wellbeing. At antenatal classes women are taught to take long deep breaths, not to help the back but to control the pain. Whenever my son has been close to tears, I've taught him to take deep breaths to help steady his emotions. Controlled breathing also helps when we are exercising — particularly when we are firming up the tummy muscles or exerting body pressure — it encourages the effort in the exercise!

Meanwhile, have you checked your posture? Here are some tips for those of you who suffer from weak backs.

TUESDAY: POSTURAL PROBLEMS

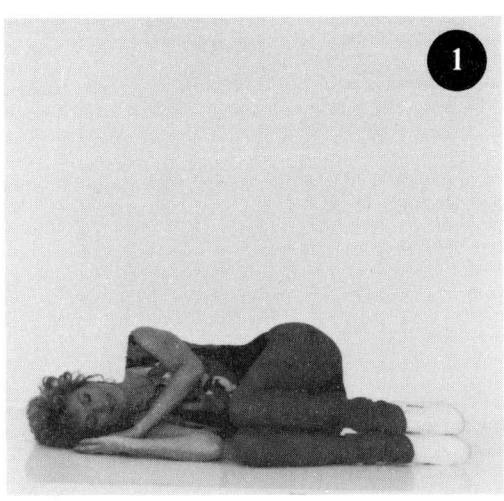

1 When lying down, draw up both knees so that the spine relaxes and forms a good curve.

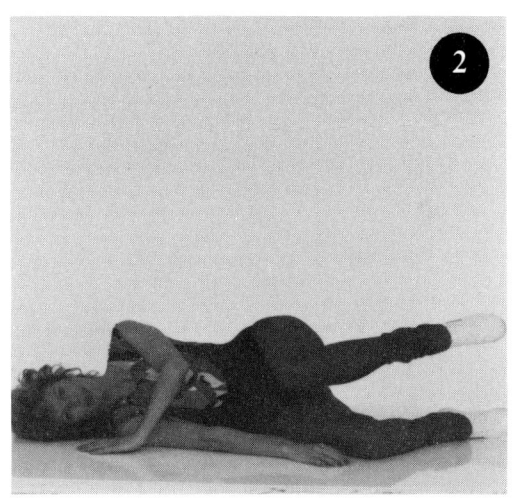

2 If you have difficulty sleeping due to back pain, try lying on your side, raise your leg and, to keep it raised, place a pillow or two between your legs.

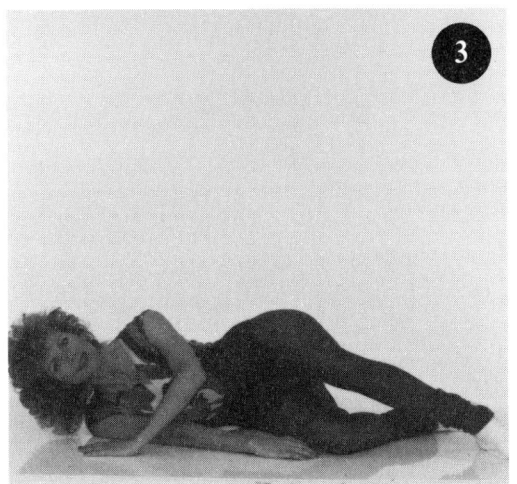

3 When you get up, come up via your side, and use your arm to help take the body weight.

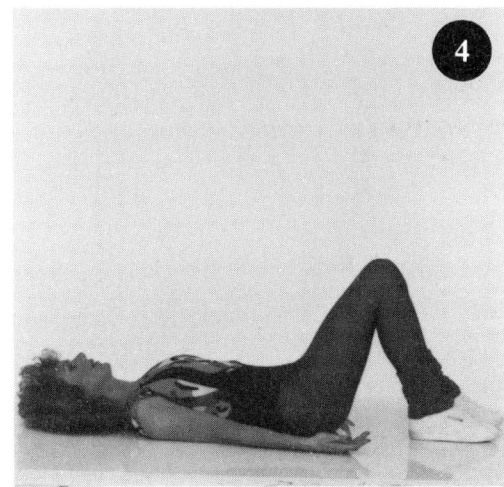

4 Tension causes more back pain, so try this position to help you relax. Lie down on the floor and draw up your knees, keeping your legs relaxed with a small gap between them. Check the small of your back is eased into the floor. Your palms should face upwards. Check that your shoulders are relaxed and practise your deep breathing. This will tense and relax the various muscles throughout your body and you will feel tense muscles 'unknot' as you breathe deeply.

TUESDAY: BACK

BACK

If you have a back problem work on the principle that you know your body best — you know your capabilities and you know your weaknesses.

If you don't have a back problem, these exercises are very important as they will strengthen up the muscles and keep the back 'free', thus helping to avoid injury.

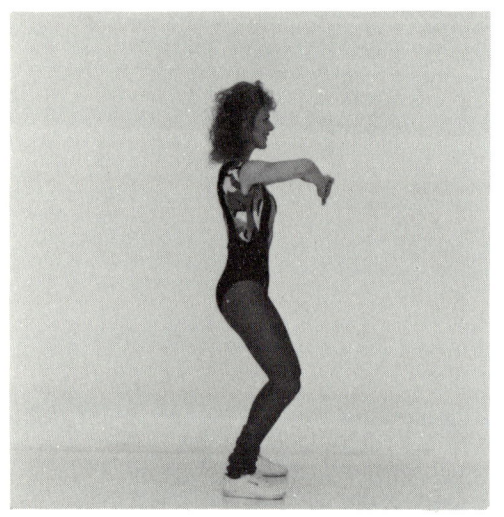

Clasp one hand over the other and bend your arms and legs. →

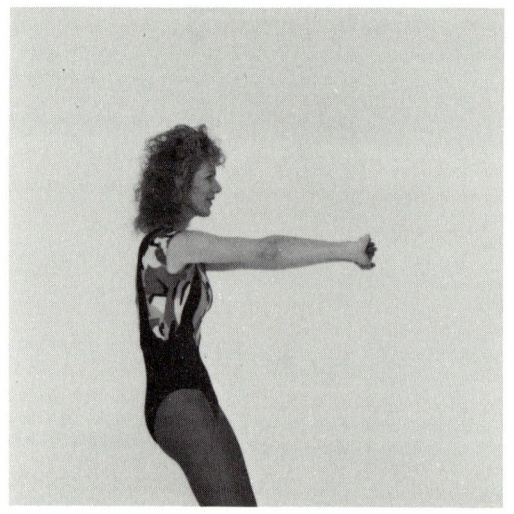

Extend your arms in front of you and, as you do so, imagine you've been hit in the stomach so that it caves in and the spine curves. →

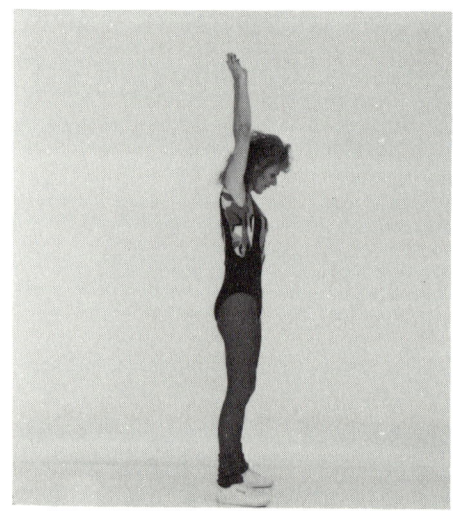

Now straighten your arms above your head stretch your legs straight and let your head go forward with your chin down towards your chest. Feel the neck extending and the back stretching. Hold that position, checking that your tummy is pulled in and that your bottom is tucked under. Repeat this exercise.

TUESDAY: BACK

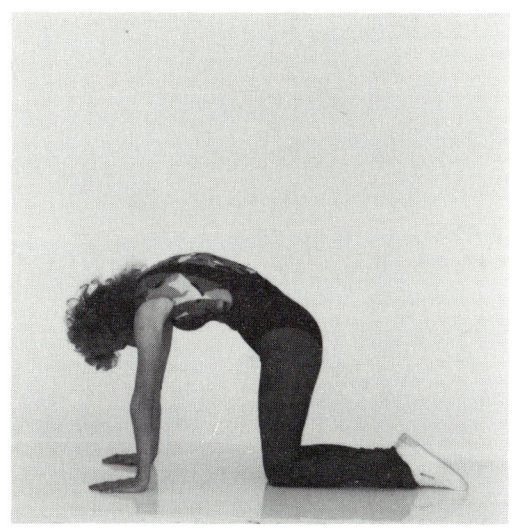 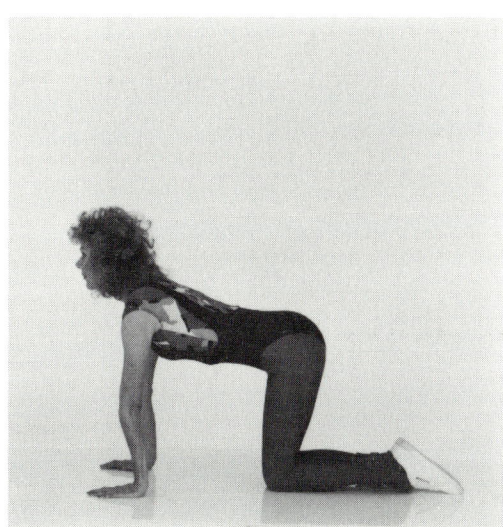 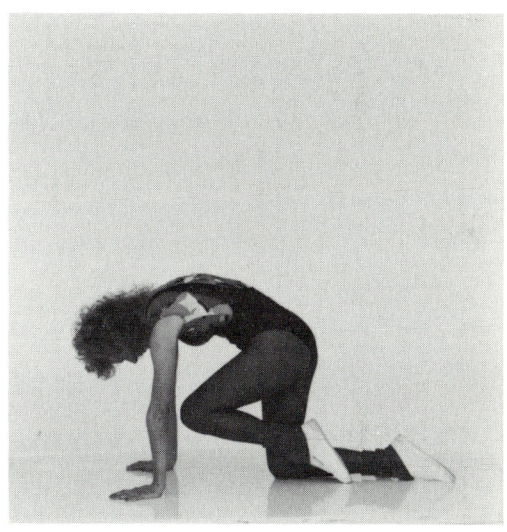

Get down on all fours, feet and legs together, palms flat on the floor. Arch your back and feel it expand, particularly across the shoulders. →

Ease the back down and reverse the stretch — flatten the back and extend your neck.

The next four movements are fluid and act as one exercise.

Crouching on all fours, bend your left knee up towards your chest. →

TUESDAY: BACK

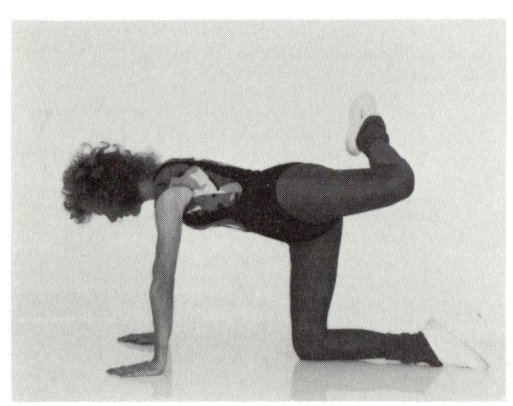 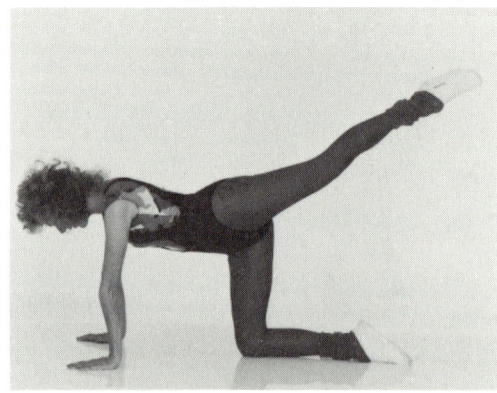 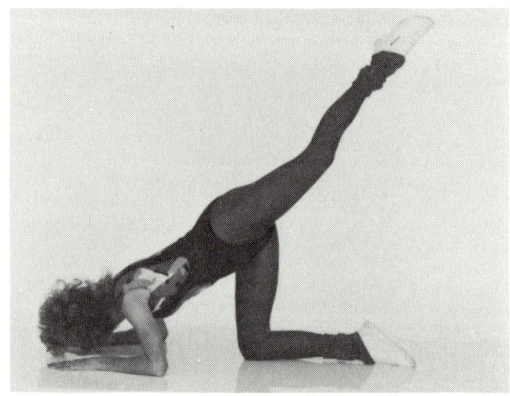

Keeping your leg bent and your back flat, take your left leg out to the side and then behind. →

Straighten your left leg out behind you →

and raise it high in the air as you drop your weight down on to your forearms. Push up through your arms and bend your leg back down to start again. Repeat two or three times and change legs.

TUESDAY: BACK

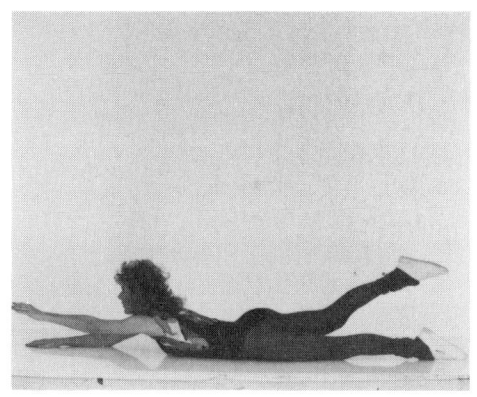 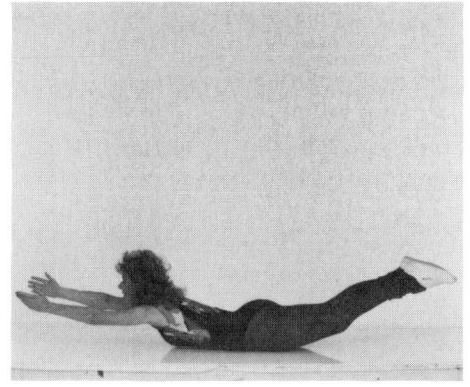 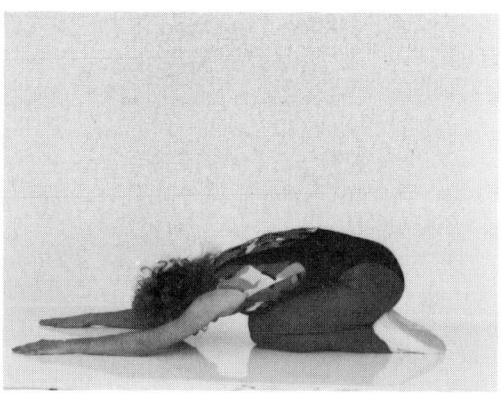

Lie down flat on the floor, head down too. Slowly raise your left arm and, at the same time, raise your right leg. Hold it, and lower. Now raise your right arm and left leg. Repeat.

Now feel as if you are flying through the air. Raise both arms, both legs and your head as high up as you can. Hold it, and lower. This exercise really strengthens up the back muscles — but don't attempt more than four at one time.

Stretch and relax by sitting your bottom back on your heels, head down, spine curved with both arms stretched out in front. Stay there, then slowly sit up through a curved spine.

TUESDAY: FACIAL EXERCISES

FACIAL EXERCISES

Our facial muscles need as much exercise as the rest of our bodies. We often try to disguise our true feelings by 'immobilizing' the muscles of the face and the stresses and strains of our everyday lives are etched upon the set expressions of our faces.

There are many contrasting exercises to firm up the face and neck muscles. It's more fun and far more revealing to do them in front of a mirror — and in private!

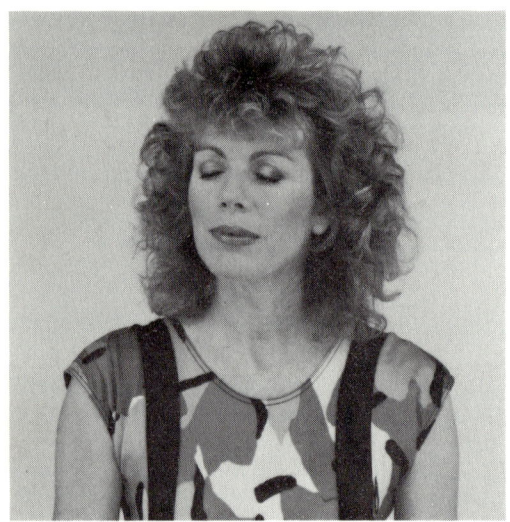
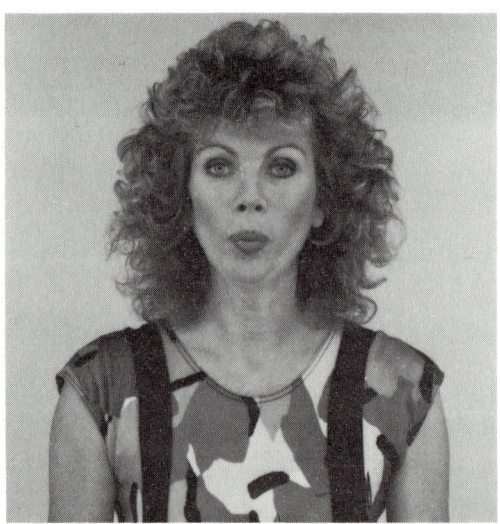
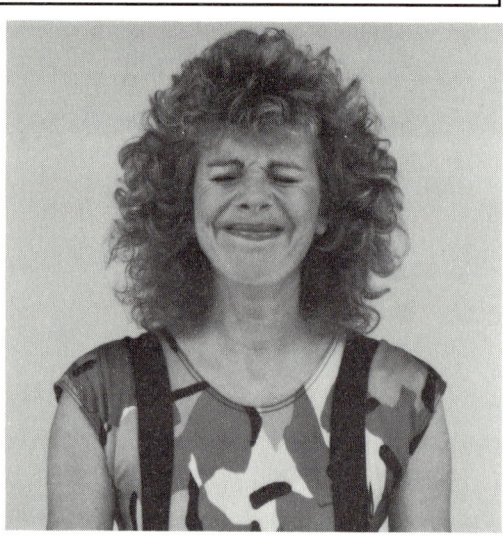

Get the lips tingling by blowing them together so that they vibrate — enjoy the sound too.

Make an exaggerated chewing motion using your lips and chin and your cheeks.

Screw your face up, frown, spread your mouth and close your eyes.

TUESDAY: FACIAL EXERCISES

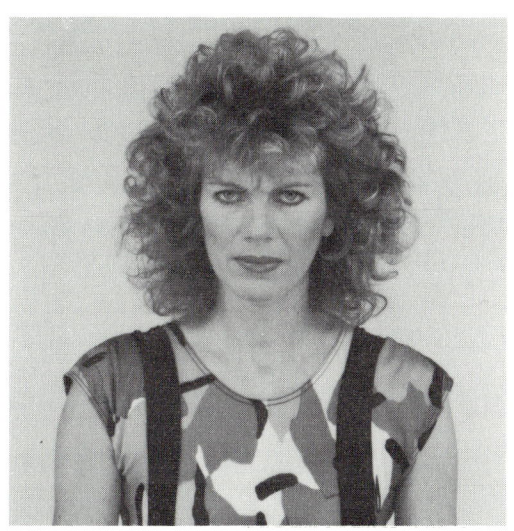

Open your eyes and frown even harder.

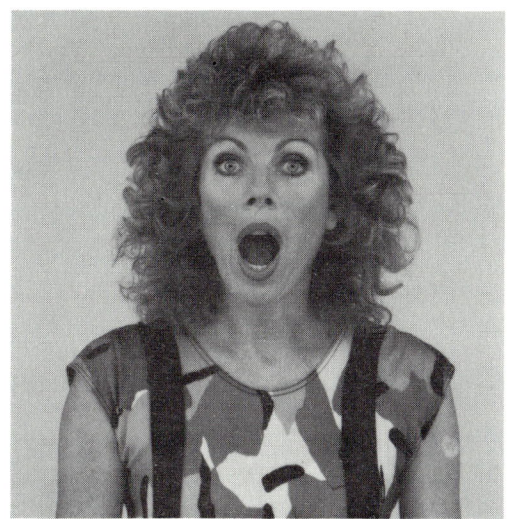

Gasp in total surprise as you open your mouth, open up your eyes — ooh!

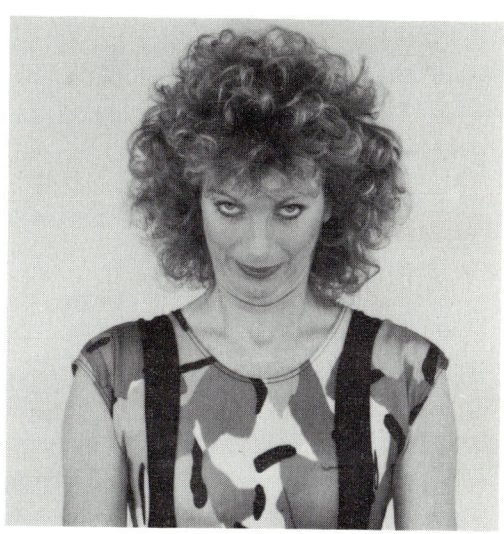

Tuck your chin in so that your jaw line is lost into the six chins!

TUESDAY: FACIAL EXERCISES

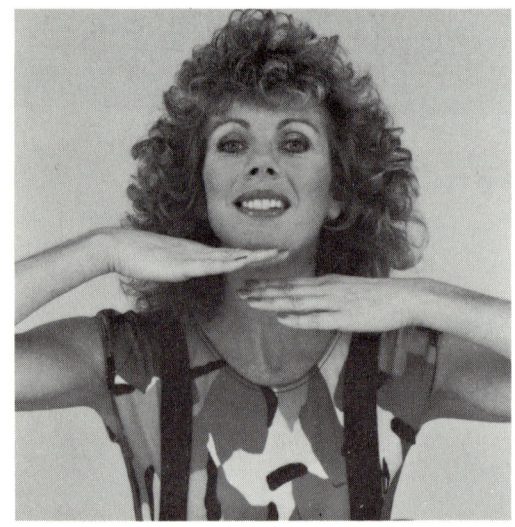 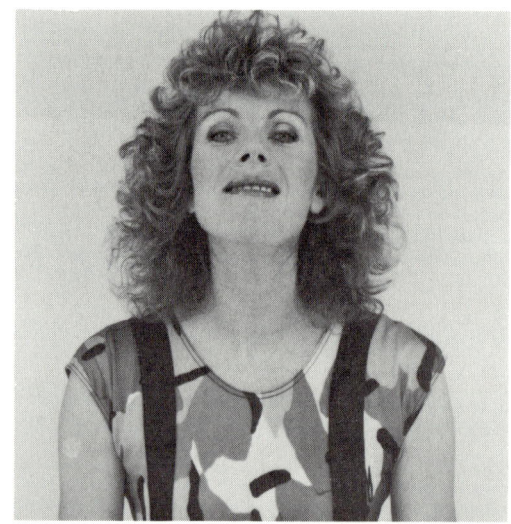 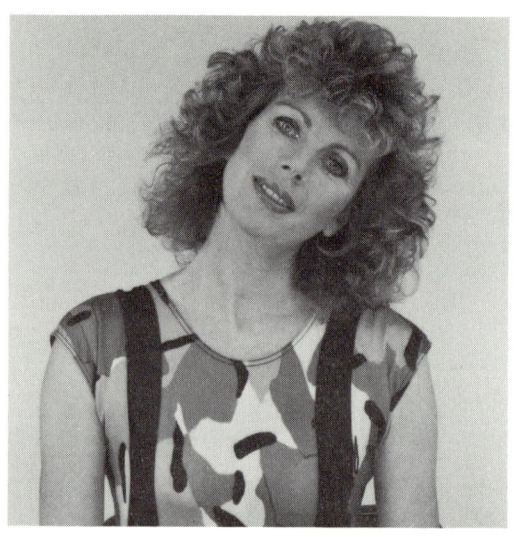

Head posture can accentuate the flabby chins around the jaw line. Keep your head erect and, in a circular movement with the hands, gently massage the flesh under the jaw. In other words, 'Chin up'!

Finish off by jutting the jaw forward, extending the chin outwards and stretching the neck.

The next exercise sequence will make you aware of the weight of the head and is good for relaxing the neck muscles.

Incline your head to your right, let it go and don't raise your shoulders. Bring your head back up. →

TUESDAY: FACIAL EXERCISES

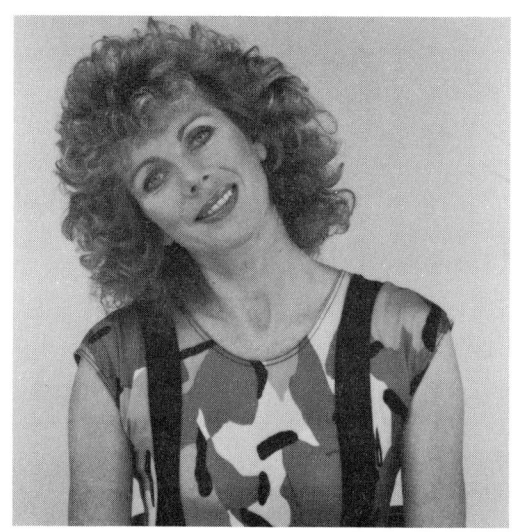

Incline your head to the left, and back to the centre. →

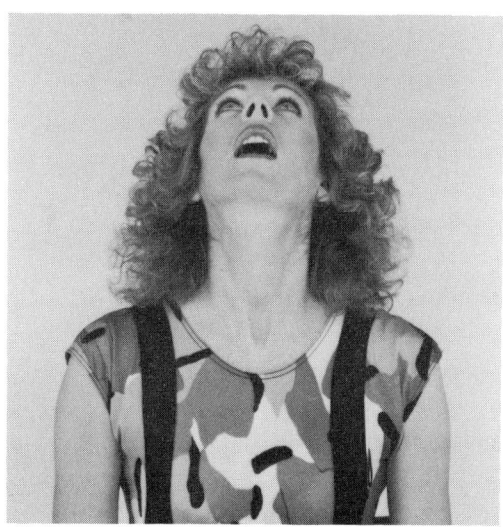

Let your head fall back and open your mouth so that you don't strain your neck. Bring your head back up to the centre. →

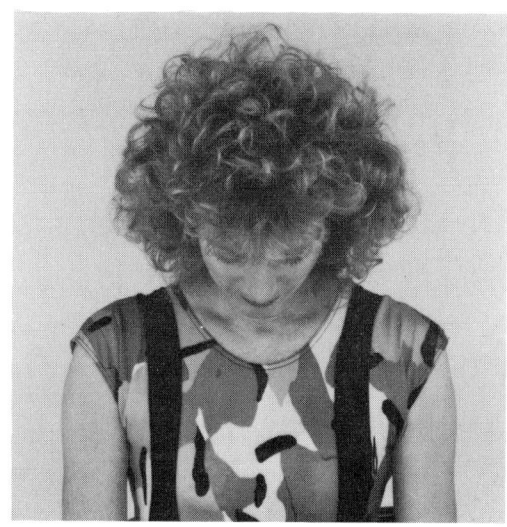

Then let your head fall forwards, chin towards your chest stretching the back of your neck. Bring it back up to the centre — and smile!

TUESDAY: HIPS, THIGHS AND BOTTOM STAGE II

HIPS, THIGHS AND BOTTOM STAGE II

On with the next stage of working on this problem area. Attempt four to eight of each exercise but, if you find them too difficult, keep working on yesterday's stage I exercises.

First of all shake out your leg muscles — rather like a runner does before the start of a race — to make sure they are relaxed.

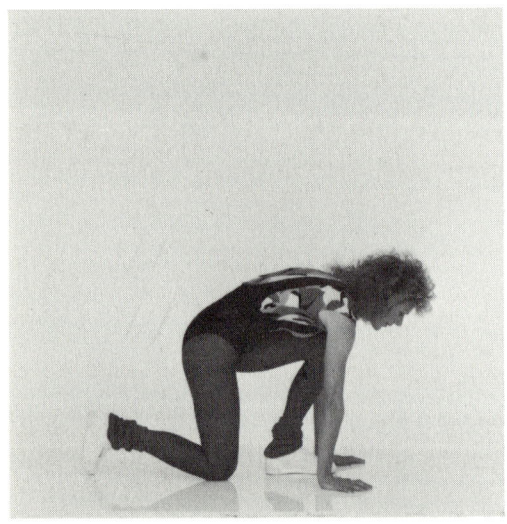

Kneel down on your right knee, left leg bent in front, foot flat on the floor and hands flat on the floor in front. →

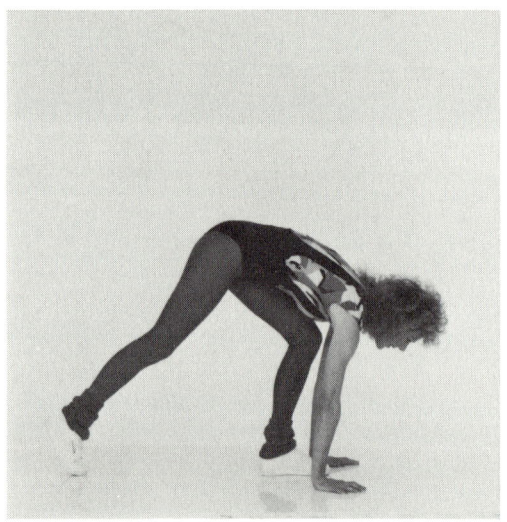

Rise up, aiming to straighten your right leg. Keep the weight on your front thigh. Imagine you are on the starting line for a race and flow these two movements together, swapping legs.

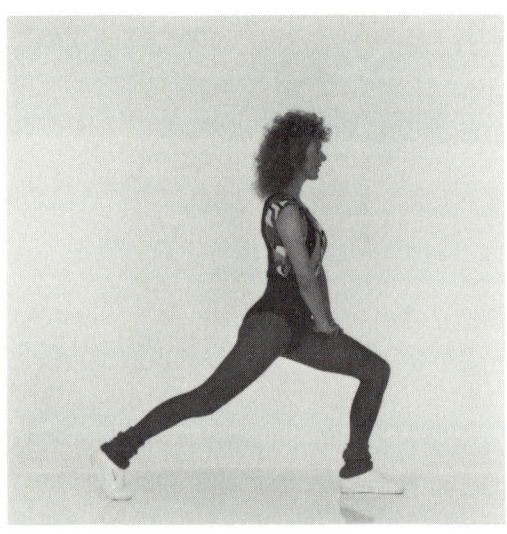

Face your right side, bend your right leg and extend your left leg out behind you. Hold this position. →

TUESDAY: HIPS, THIGHS AND BOTTOM STAGE II

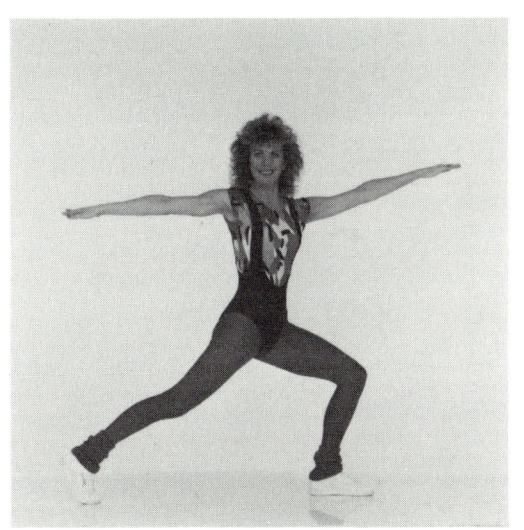 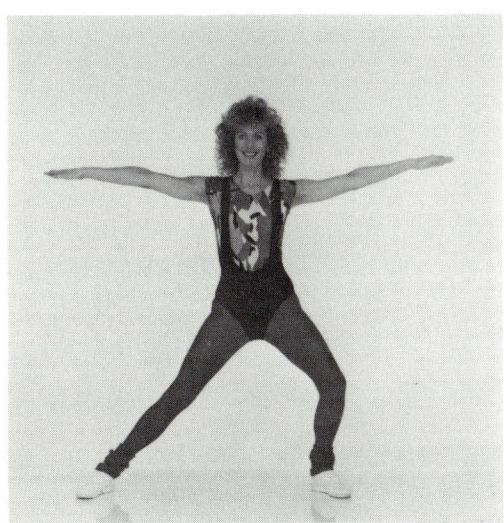 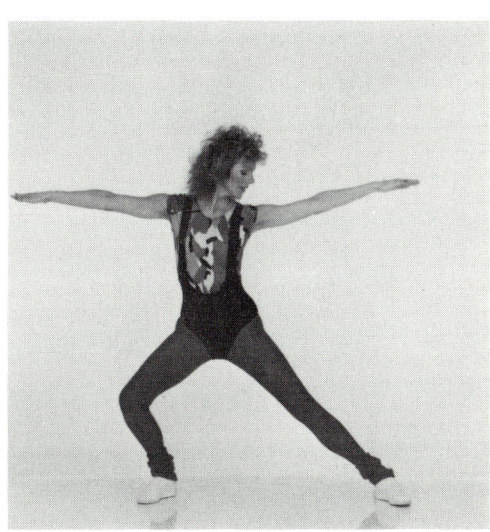

Now turn from your waist — keeping your weight on the front thigh — and raise your arms out to the side. →

Face the front, bend your right leg and stretch your left leg by keeping your left foot flat on the floor, toes facing front. →

Transfer the weight by bending your left leg and straightening your right leg, keeping the toes facing front. Repeat this sequence and change sides.

TUESDAY: HIPS, THIGHS AND BOTTOM STAGE II

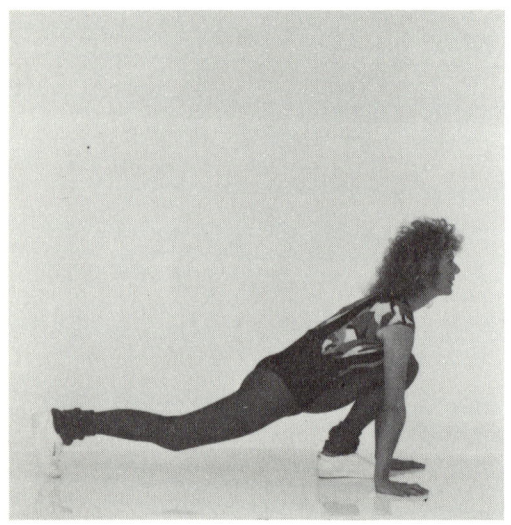 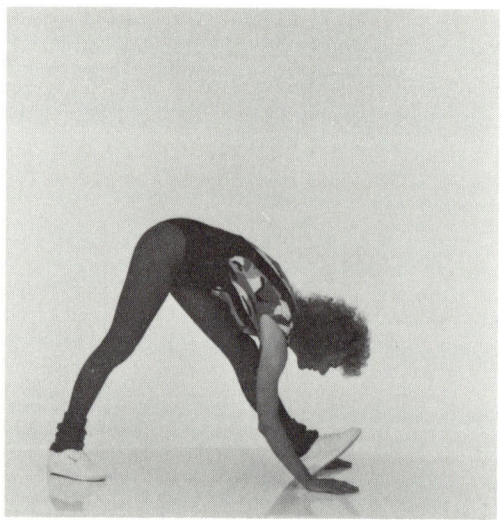 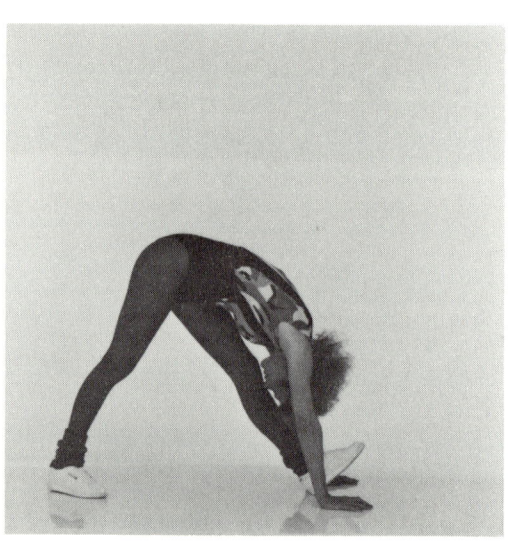

Crouch down on the floor keeping your left leg near your chest with the left foot and both hands flat on the floor, and extend your right leg out behind you. →

Transfer your weight by straightening your left leg as you rise up and reach over a straight leg. To get an even greater leg stretch, raise the toes of your front foot. →

Only when you have achieved this position can you aim to touch your knee with your nose! Practise again and change sides.

TUESDAY: HIPS, THIGHS AND BOTTOM STAGE II

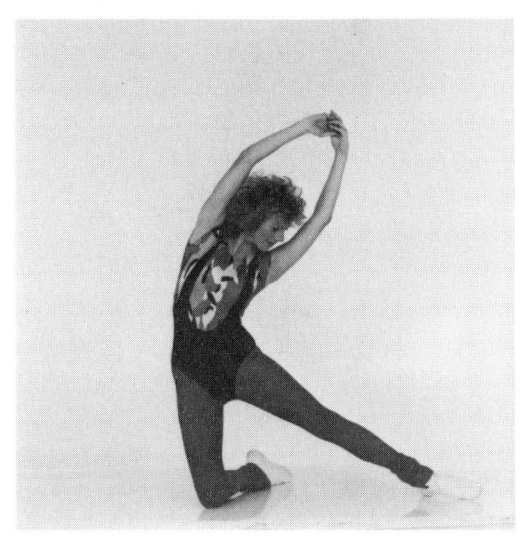 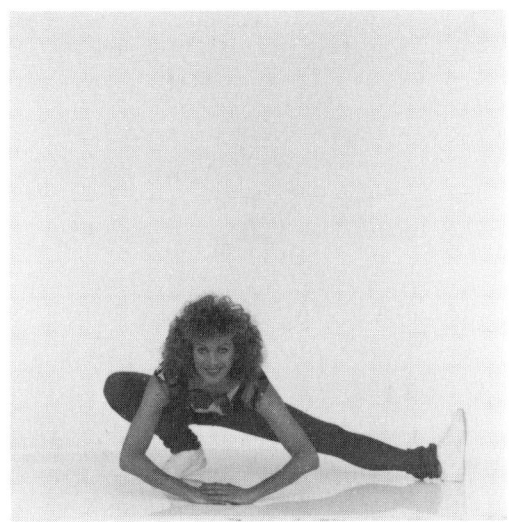 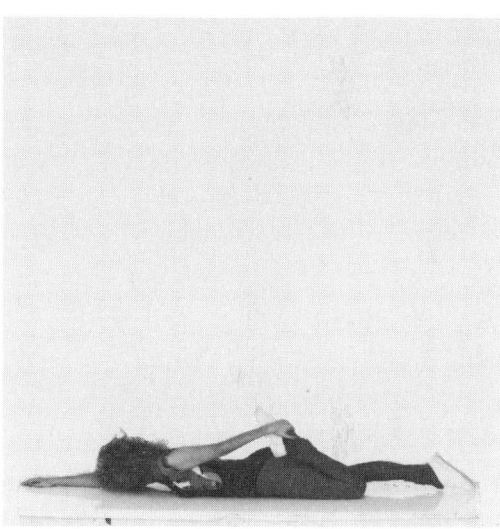

Kneel on your left leg and extend your right leg out to the side. Clasp your hands above your head and curve over towards your right thigh. Repeat and change sides.

Bend your left leg and straighten your right leg out to the side, toes pointing upwards. Flatten your back as you reach forward, hands on the floor. Keep your left knee pointing to the side. Change legs.

Lie face down on the floor and grasp your left foot with your left hand. Don't pull at it or keep stretching the thigh, just hold it. Change sides.

Wednesday

> **WARM UP**
> Each exercise should be attempted eight times. Remember to adjust your position if anything hurts or twinges — it could be that your body is simply wrongly placed for the exercise. If you still experience pain then leave that particular exercise out.

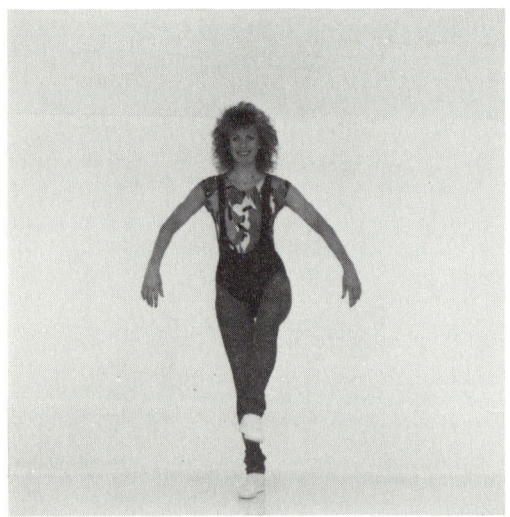

Loosely shake out the body. Make sure you are relaxed and warm.

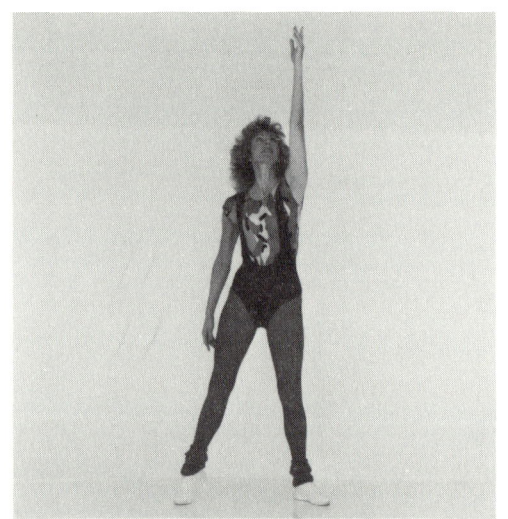

Stand with your legs and feet a comfortable distance apart, and raise your right arm and your left heel at the same time. Reach right up then lower your arm, making a fist at the side of your body, bend the elbow and lower the left heel. Continue to raise and lower arm and heel eight times and repeat on your left side.

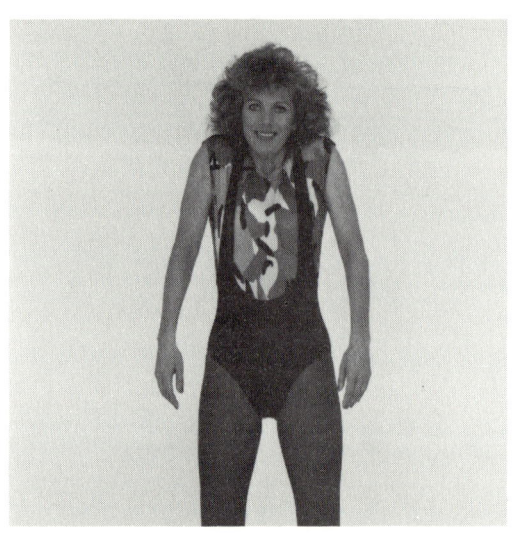

Loosely shrug both shoulders up towards your ears. Hold them there and lower them. Continue this movement up and down — as if saying 'I don't know!'.

WEDNESDAY: WARM UP

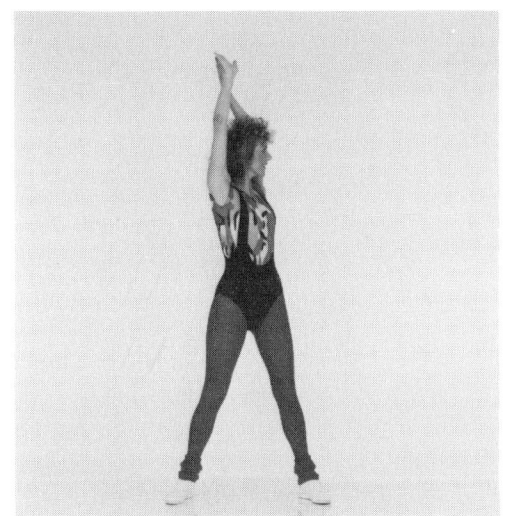
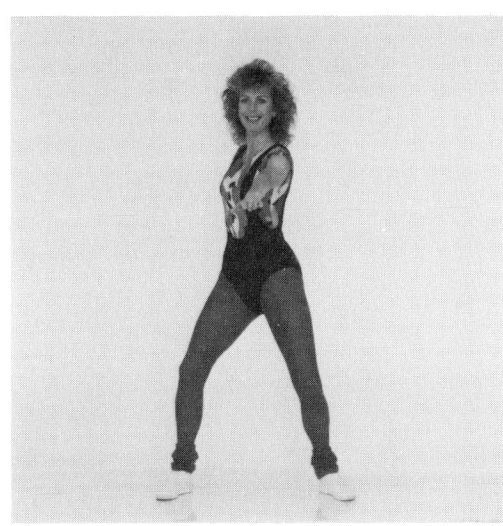
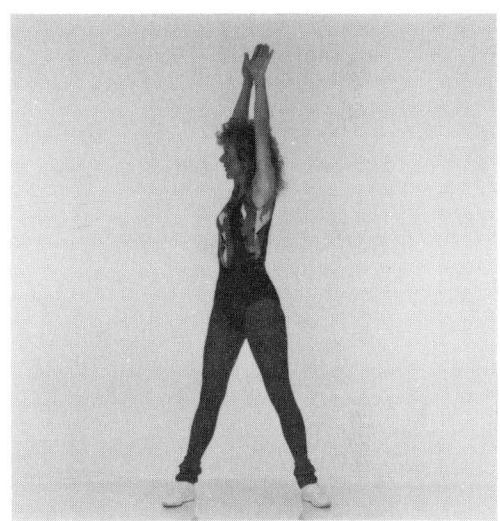

Turn from the waist to look to your right. As you do so, raise both arms out to the sides and up over your head. →

Lower them down by your sides as you bend the legs and face front to. →

Swing them up above your head while turning to face your left side. Lower them down again, face the front and bend your legs to continue the exercise flow.

WEDNESDAY: WARM UP

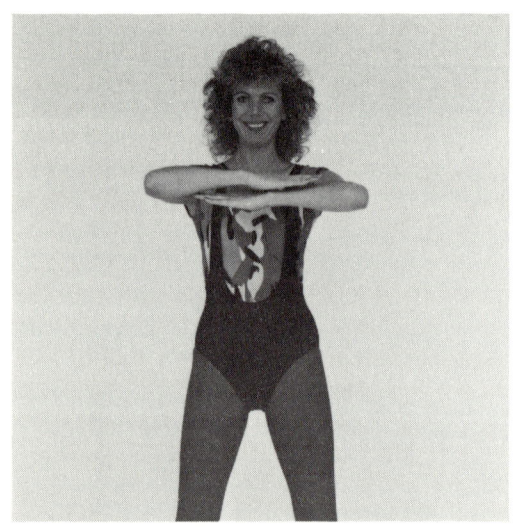 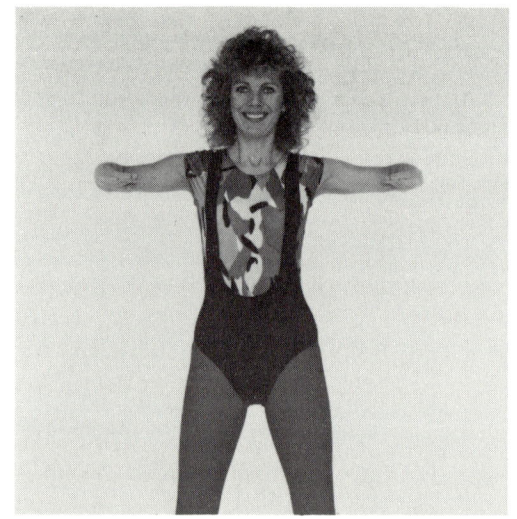 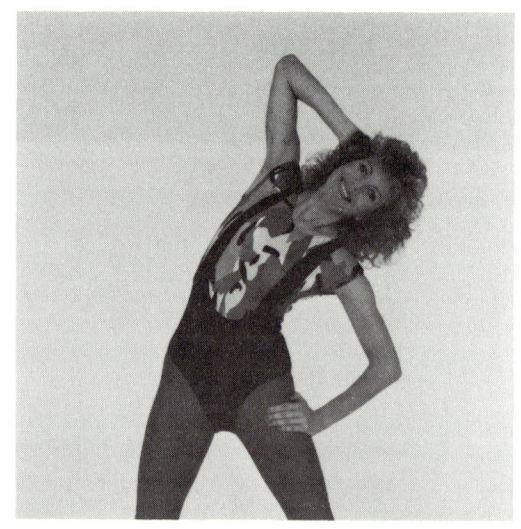

Raise both arms in front of you, bent at the elbows, chest height, one arm over the other — not touching. Keep your shoulders down. →

Keeping your upper arms straight, ease your arms back — without any jerking movement. Feel the shoulder blades squeeze together behind you. Bring your arms back to the front.

Relax your knees. Place your right hand at the top of your right thigh and your left hand at the side of your head. Lean over to your right so that your left elbow is pointing towards the ceiling. Hold that position. Come up, change hands and lean to your left.

WEDNESDAY: WARM UP

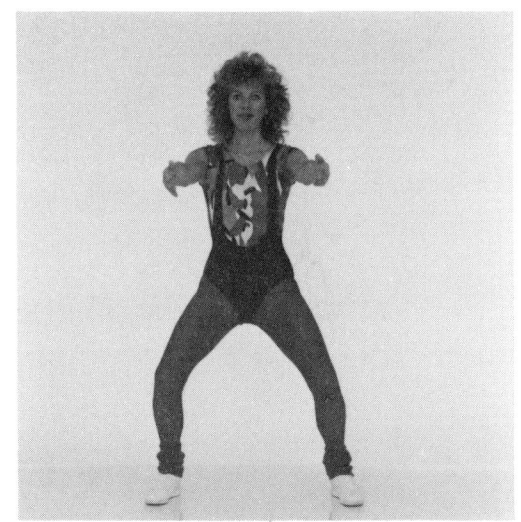
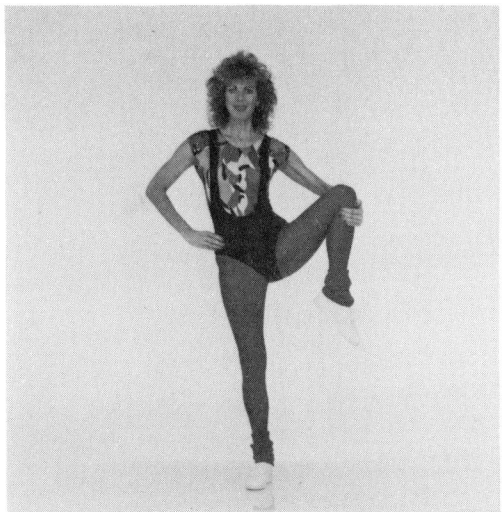
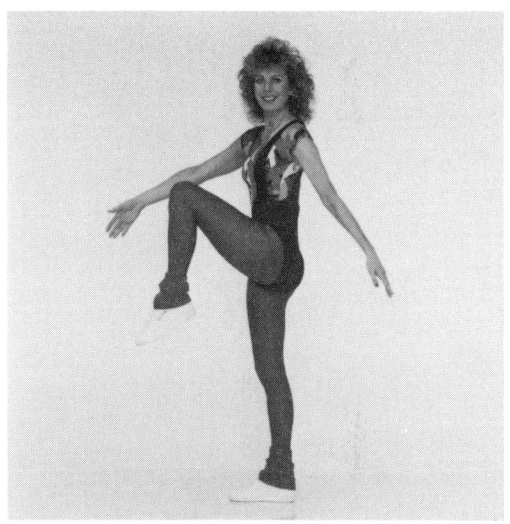

Standing with legs and feet apart, toes facing front, bend both legs, keeping the feet flat on the floor. Stretch both arms out in front and hold that position. Straighten your legs. You might only be able to do this three or four times to begin with.

Balance on your left leg and raise your right knee out to your right side — turning out from the very top of your leg. Hold it below the knee and try to ease the leg up, then lower your leg back down. Repeat with your left leg.

Finish your warm up by high marching on the spot or around the room. Raise each knee as high as possible and swing your arms — feel those thighs working!

Shake out and relax the muscles.

WEDNESDAY: CHAIR EXERCISES

CHAIR EXERCISES

Chair exercises play a very important part of an exercise programme. If you have problems with balance or suffer particularly from hip and knee problems then this set of exercises is ideal for you.

Likewise, if you are substantially overweight, gentle exercise in a chair will put less strain on your heart.

Do not underestimate the value of these exercises: you can do almost all of Monday's waist exercises from a chair! If you suffer from ME or arthritis, then chair exercises will encourage you to keep working your body.

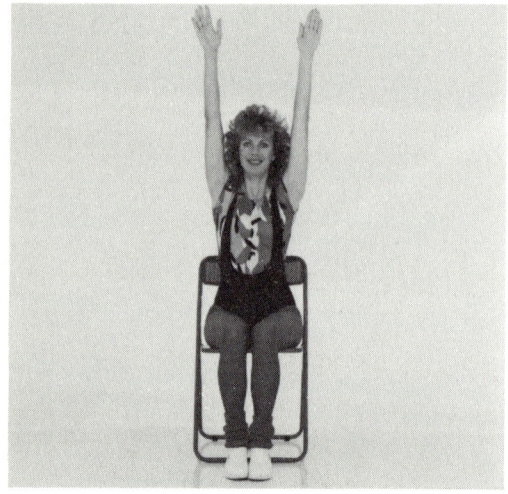

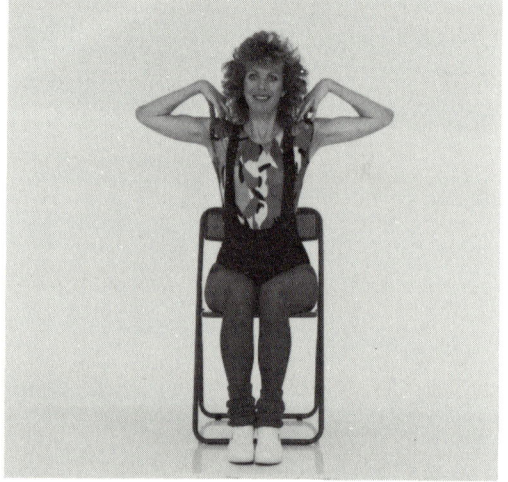

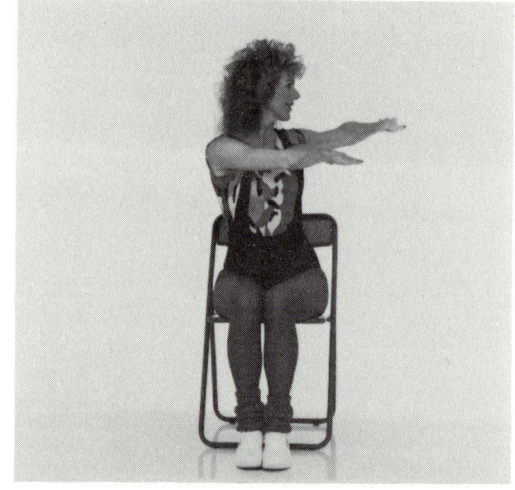

Have a good stretch and reach up to fill that space.

Place your hands on your shoulders and, guided by your elbows, circle your shoulders up and round. Reverse the circle.

Bend your left arm in front of you at chest height. Extend your right arm to the side and, turning from the waist, ease your torso round to the right. Bring your arms back to the front and reverse the exercise, bending your right arm, extending your left and turning to your left.

WEDNESDAY: CHAIR EXERCISES

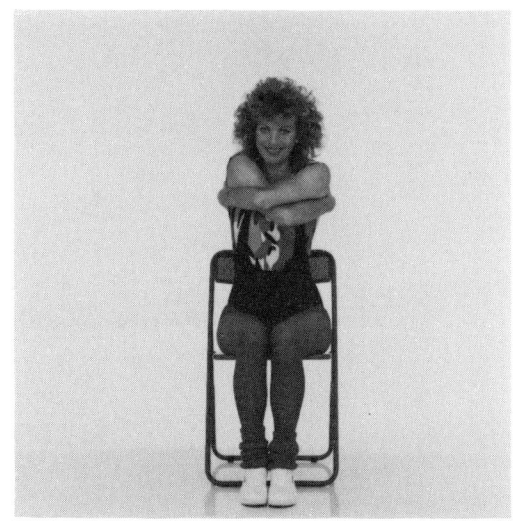

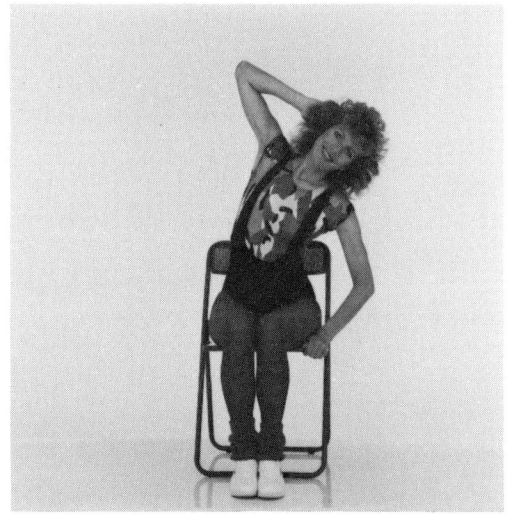

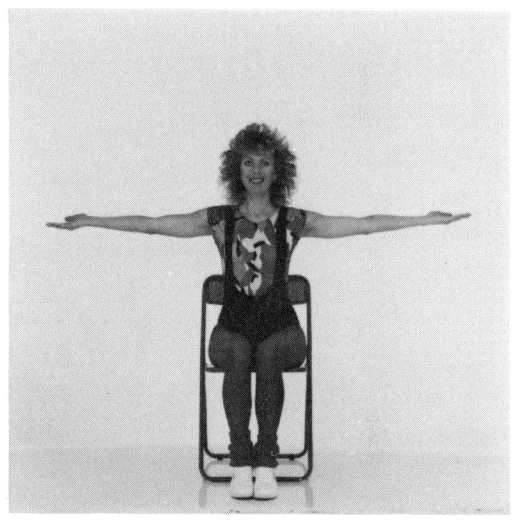

Hug yourself! Wrap your arms around your body, shoulders up. Unfold and try again: see how far you can reach round with your fingertips.

Place your right hand on the side of the chair for balance. Place your left hand at the side of your head, elbow up to the ceiling. Lean directly over to your right. Centralize, change hands and lean to your left.

Stretch both arms out to your sides and, with a twisting movement, turn both arms up and over. Keep your arms straight.

WEDNESDAY: CHAIR EXERCISES

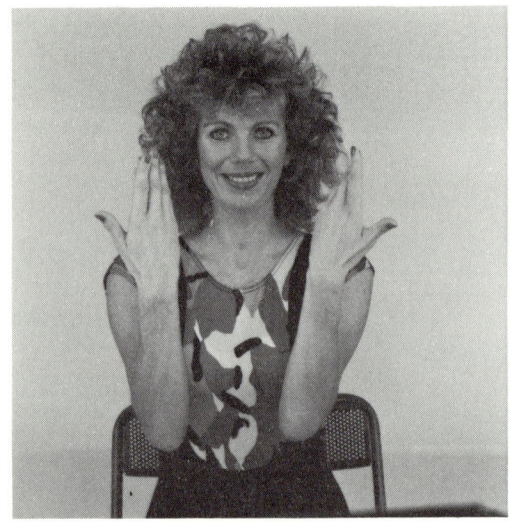

Bend your arms in front of you, elbows down, and circle both hands round away from each other and then back.

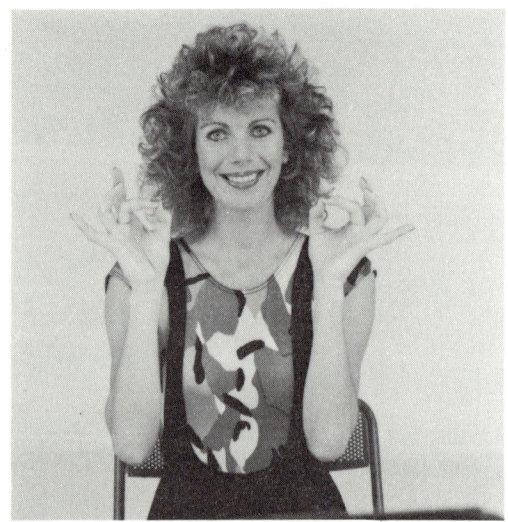

Touch your thumb with each finger — the tip of the finger should touch the tip of your thumb. Do this continuously, working from the little finger to the index finger and out again.

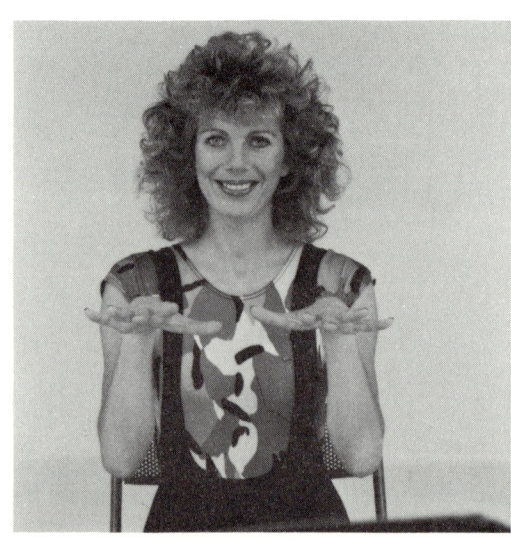

With both hands in front of you, palms down, make a fist, then splay the fingers out, spreading and stretching them, and make a fist again.

WEDNESDAY: CHAIR EXERCISES

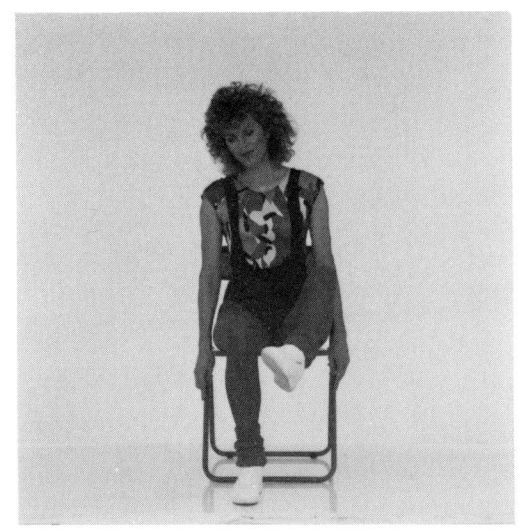 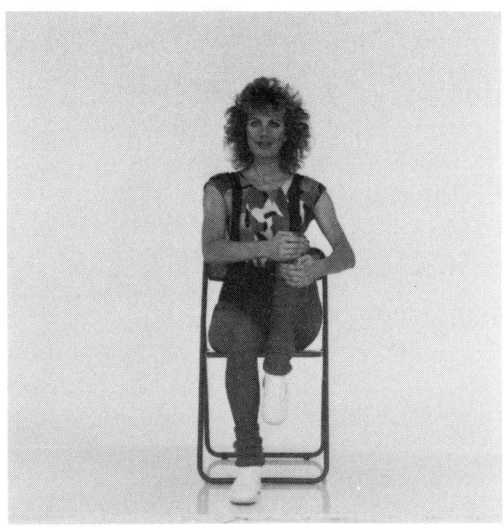 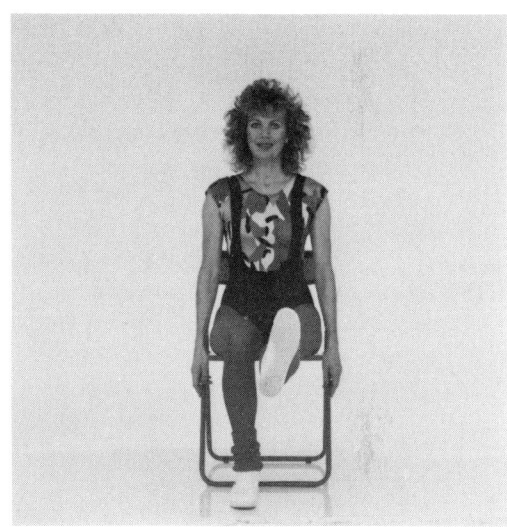

Raise your right foot and draw large, continuous circles in the air, clockwise and anticlockwise. Change feet.

Hug your right knee, holding it just below the knee, and ease it up. →

Extend the leg straight in front, foot up, toes pointing to the ceiling, and lower. Repeat and change feet.

WEDNESDAY: ARMS AND SHOULDERS

ARMS AND SHOULDERS

Help relax the tension of the week by squeezing out the 'weight of the world' that sits squarely upon your shoulders! Tension in this area causes back pain, bad posture and headaches. Strengthen the shoulders and square up to the world!

The arm muscles are an overworked part of the body's engine and they need constant toning. This is also an area that women worry about, as flabby upper arms can look very unsightly. So, every Wednesday, work at the following exercises and develop your muscle tone.

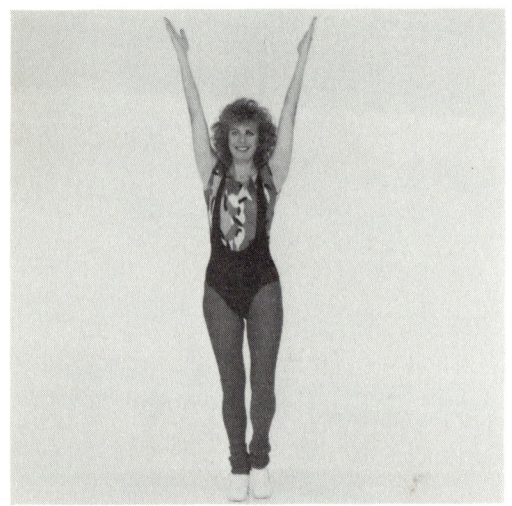

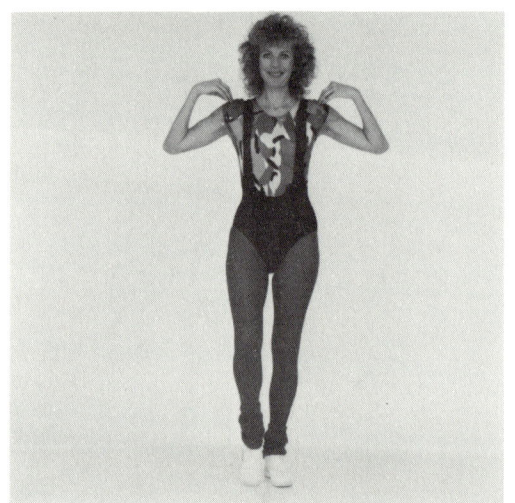

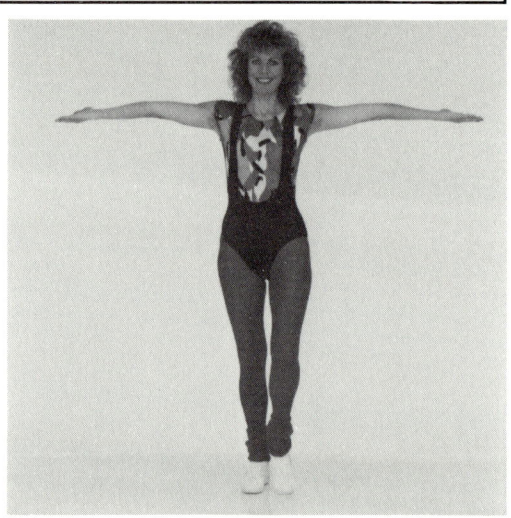

The following sequence of four movements can either be done standing or lightly marching on the spot — almost as a jog.

Raise both arms straight up. →

On the next beat, bring your hands on to your shoulders, touching with your fingertips. →

Extend both arms out to your sides, palms facing towards the ceiling. →

WEDNESDAY: ARMS AND SHOULDERS

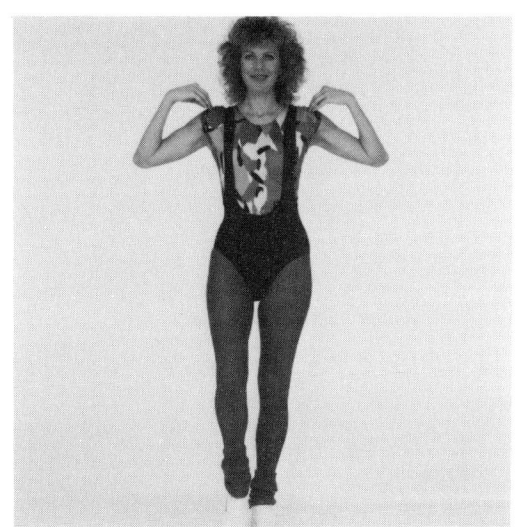 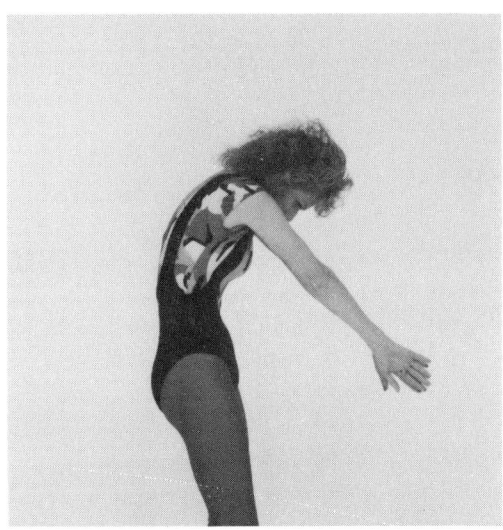 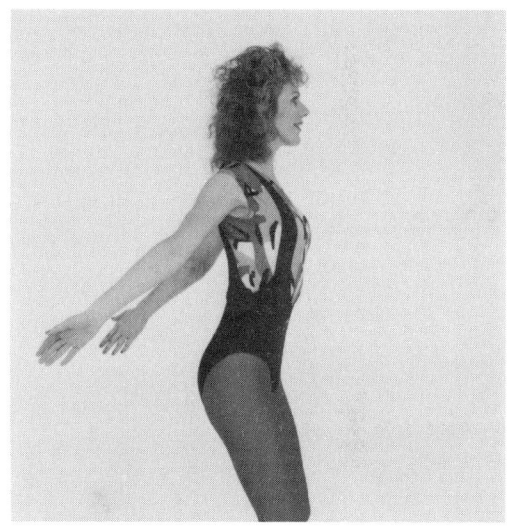

Bring both arms back to your shoulders and repeat the pattern.

Let both arms fall forwards — your shoulders will rise up as you do this. Curve your spine and touch the backs of your hands together. →

Open both arms up, taking them to the sides and behind. As the spine straightens the chest opens and the shoulders relax down. This exercise must be done slowly and smoothly.

WEDNESDAY: ARMS AND SHOULDERS

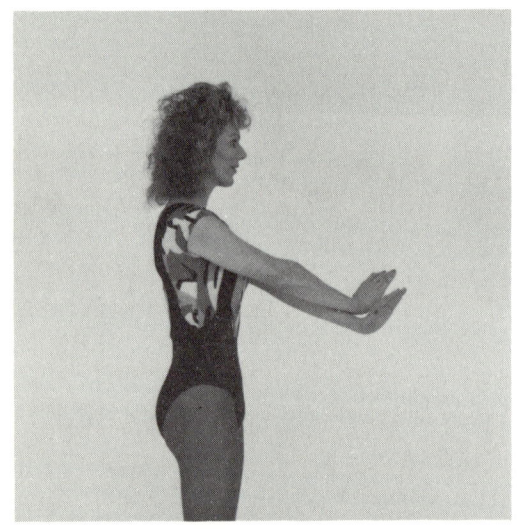

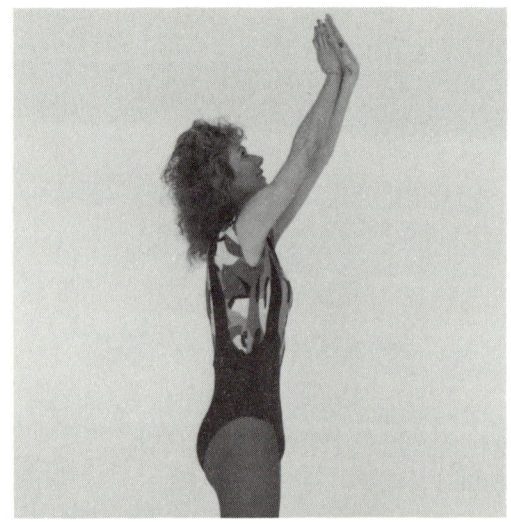

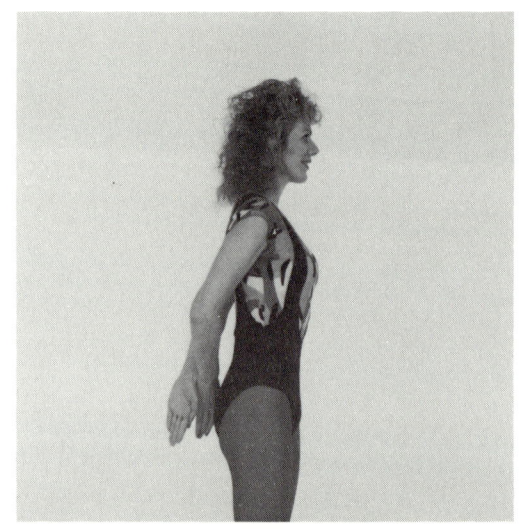

Cross both arms in front of you, keeping them straight, with your palms and fingers pointing to the ceiling. Starting low, criss-cross each arm over the other in small, tight movements. →

Continue this, raising both arms as high as you can, then bring them down in the same way.

This time cross your arms behind your back. Keep them as straight as possible and repeat the tight, criss-crossing movement. Your hands should be flat and arms should be kept close together.

WEDNESDAY: ARMS AND SHOULDERS

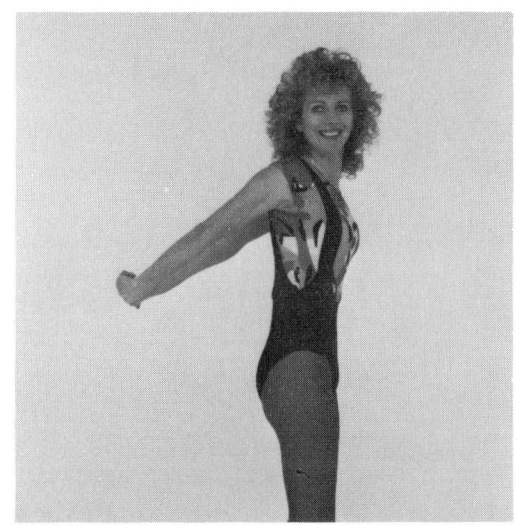 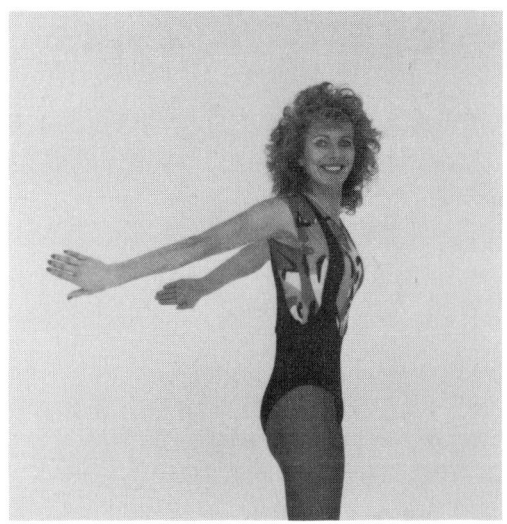 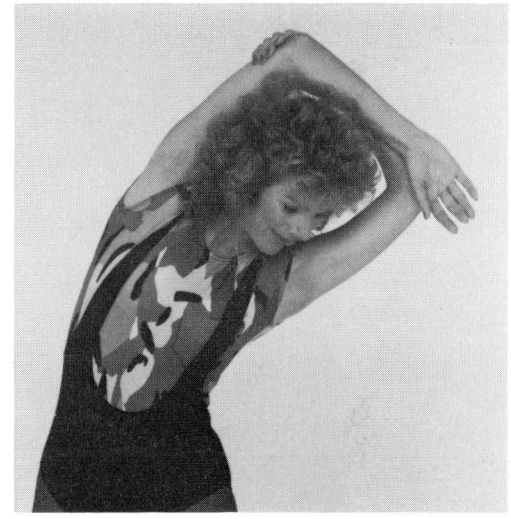

Clasp your hands behind your back. Keeping your arms straight, raise them as high as you can. Hold them there, and slowly lower. Repeat.

Raise you arms behind you as high as you can. Keep them at that height and squeeze them in and out with a minimal movement.

To finally loosen the shoulders, raise both arms above your head and bend them over, holding your left elbow with your right hand. Lean to your right side and apply pressure to your left arm to stretch and reach over. Change sides, holding your right elbow with your left hand and repeat.

WEDNESDAY: HIPS, THIGHS AND BOTTOM STAGE III

HIPS, THIGHS AND BOTTOM STAGE III

Down we go to tone-up the 'pear-shaped' area! Hips help define the female form, but drooping buttocks and flabby thighs are not a pretty sight. Some of these floor exercises are difficult, but take your time. See how many you can comfortably achieve with each of these toning exercises. Always relax your leg muscles at both the start and finish of the exercise sequence.

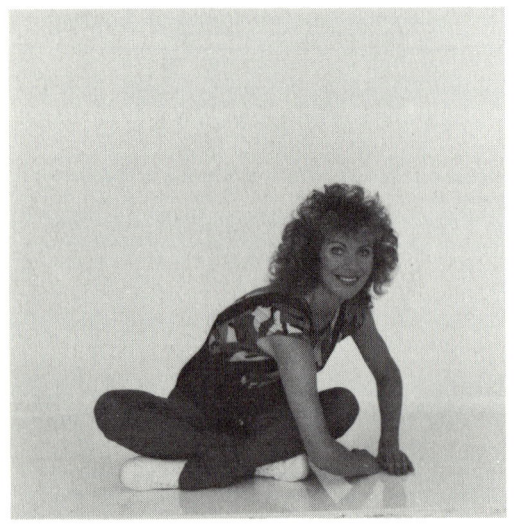

Sit cross-legged on the floor, letting the knees fall outwards. Turning from your waist, place (or attempt to!) both hands flat on the floor to your right. →

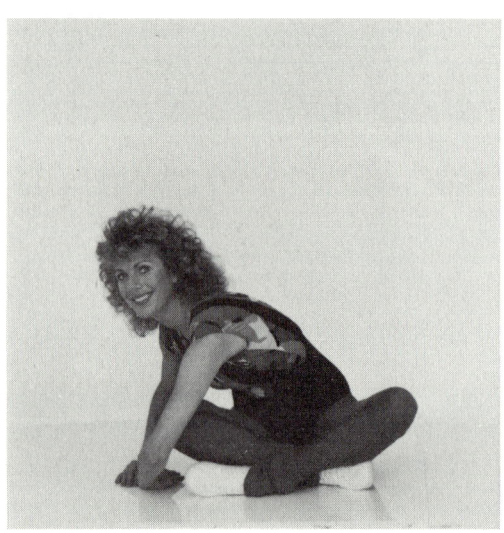

Sit up and repeat the exercise to your left.

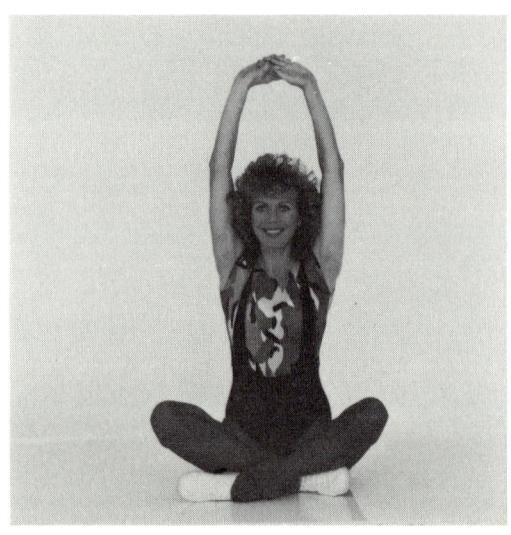

Still sitting cross-legged, clasp both hands above your head and hold that stretch.

WEDNESDAY: HIPS, THIGHS AND BOTTOM STAGE III

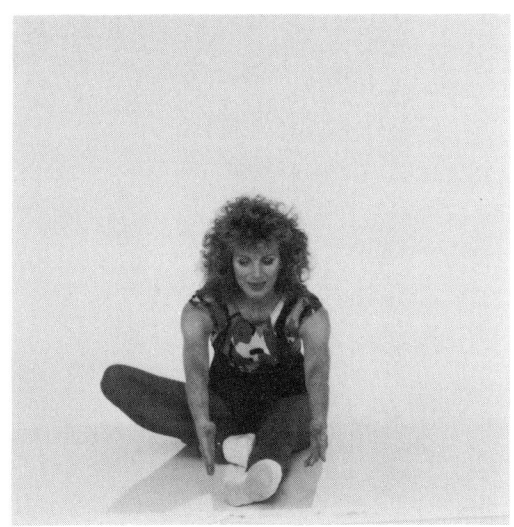

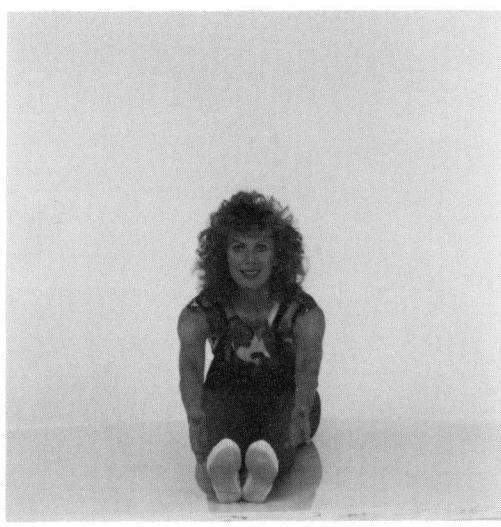

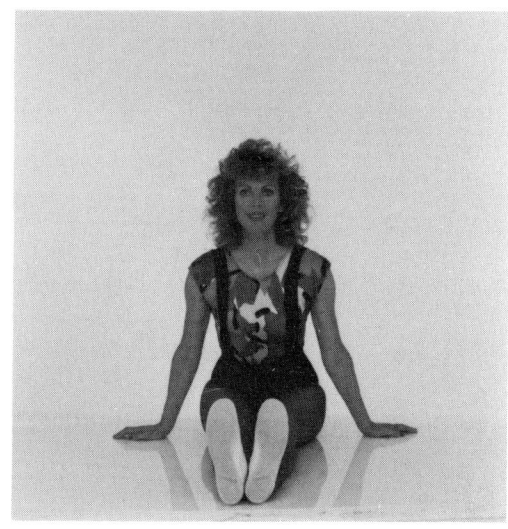

Place your right leg straight in front of you on the floor. Bend your left leg so that your left foot is flat against the inside of your right thigh, knee out. Gently reach forward, easing out of the back of the right leg. Change sides.

With both legs outstretched, gently reach forward, toes pointing down.

This time, point both feet up to the ceiling and place your hands either side on the floor. Keep your back straight as you ease your torso forward and keep upright.

WEDNESDAY: HIPS, THIGHS AND BOTTOM STAGE III

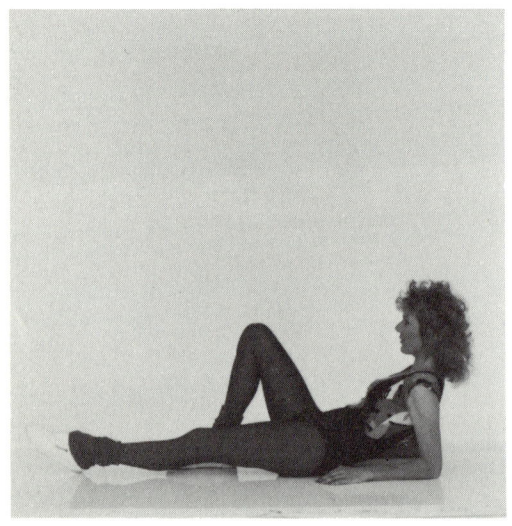

Lie back on your elbows. Bend your right leg, keeping the foot flat on the floor. →

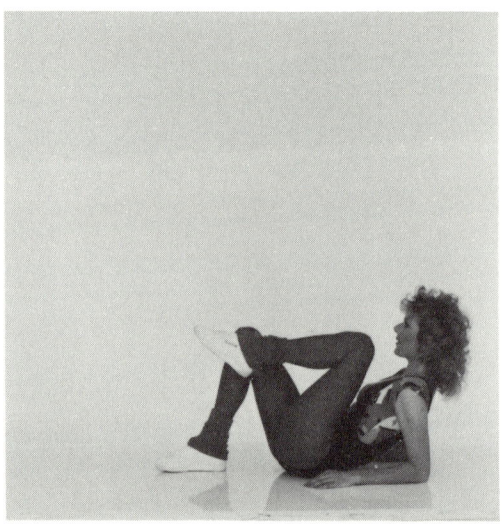

Bend your left knee back towards your chin. →

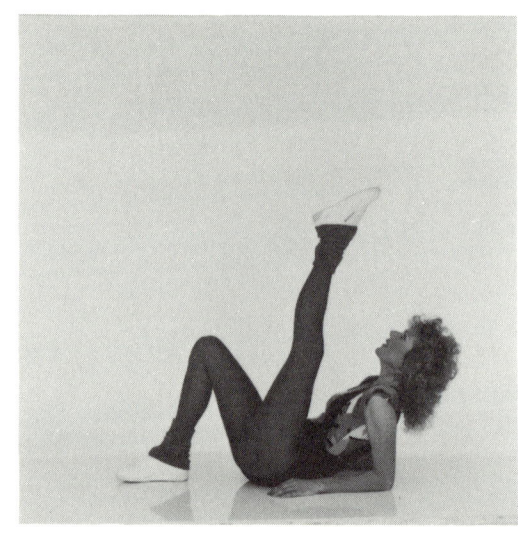

Then lower your left leg straight back down on to the floor, and kick it straight up in the air. Lower. Repeat these movements and change legs.

WEDNESDAY: HIPS, THIGHS AND BOTTOM STAGE III

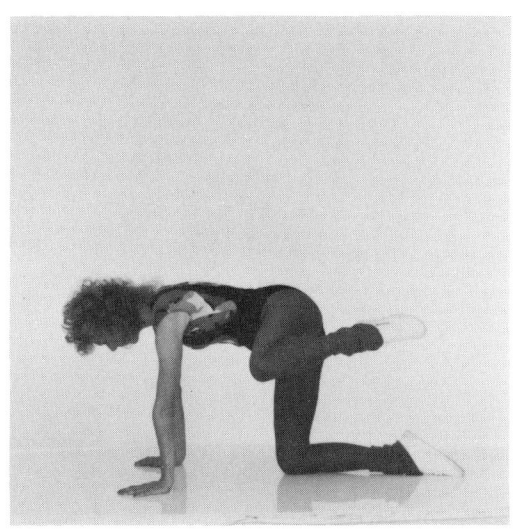 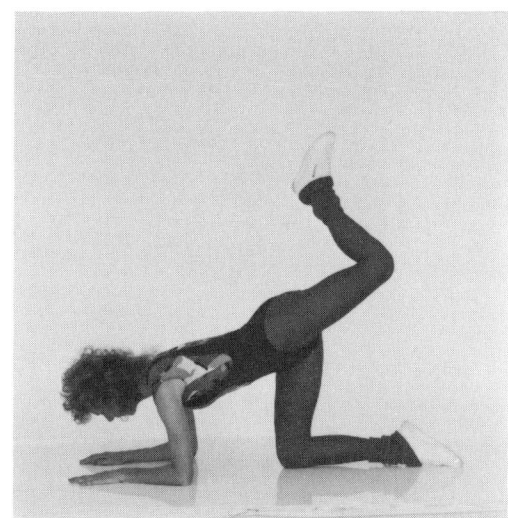 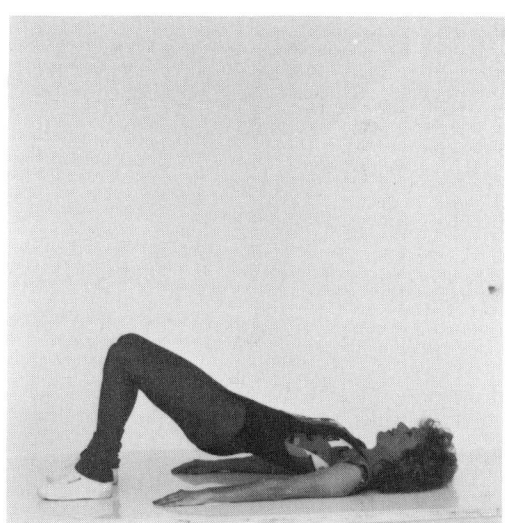

This is called the 'cock-a-leg' — for obvious reasons! Get down on all fours. Bend your left leg out to your side, raise it as high as you can, keeping it bent, and bring it back in. Change legs and repeat.

Still down on all fours, lower yourself down on to your elbows. Keeping your left leg bent take it as high as you can up behind you. When you bring it back down, keep your knee off the floor. Repeat and change legs. If you feel that this puts too much strain on your back, then leave this exercise out.

Lie flat on your back, knees bent and a small distance apart. Tilt your pelvis but *don't* arch your back as you lift your bottom off the floor. Hold that position and tense the muscles in your buttocks. Relax back into the floor. Repeat.

Thursday: Stamina Day

The heart is the largest muscle in your body, and to help it pump the blood around the body efficiently you need to get your circulation going. On Stamina Day we'll do just that! These exercises flow together as one long sequence, they will exercise your cardiovascular system and speed up your metabolic rate. You will feel your heart beating faster and may feel slightly breathless after 10–15 minutes. See how much you can do: if you are not used to regular exercise only attempt the first 24 movements. This workout will certainly take you longer than eight minutes but it is essential to build up your stamina and look after your heart. Attempt each exercise eight times.

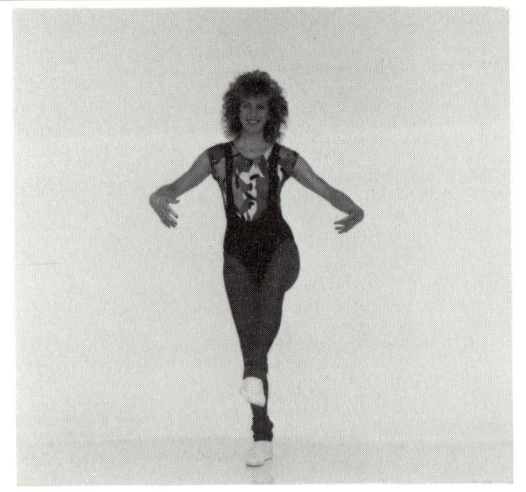

'Shake out' to relax the muscles, loosely shake out the arms, hands and shoulders, followed by the legs and feet.

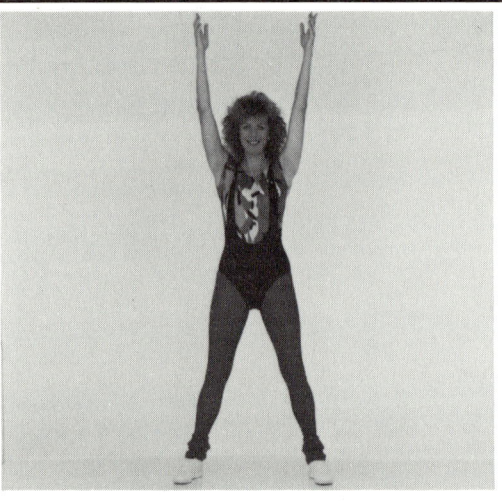

Stand tall, feet and legs apart, arms raised above your head. →

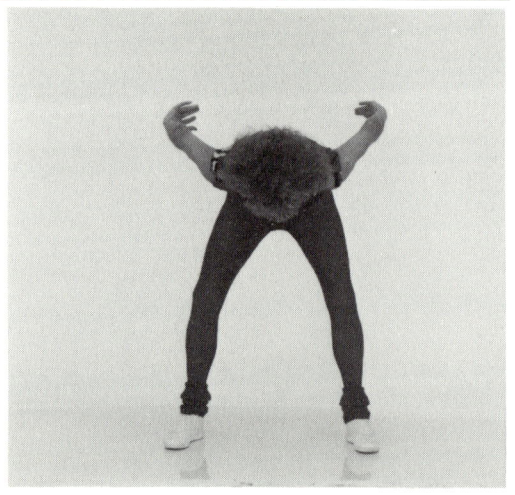

Bend your legs, as in skiing. As you do so, swing your arms down and behind. Now swing back and straighten up.

THURSDAY: STAMINA DAY

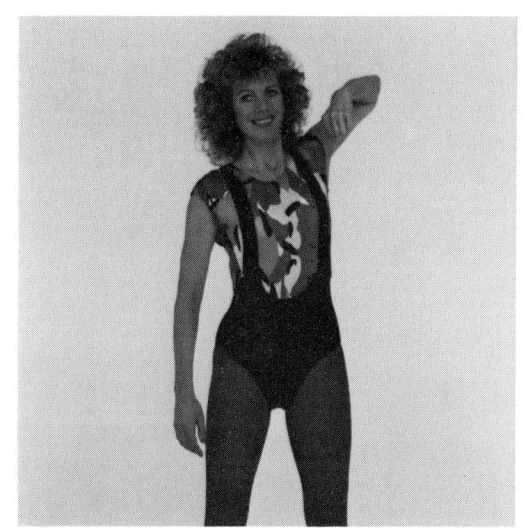 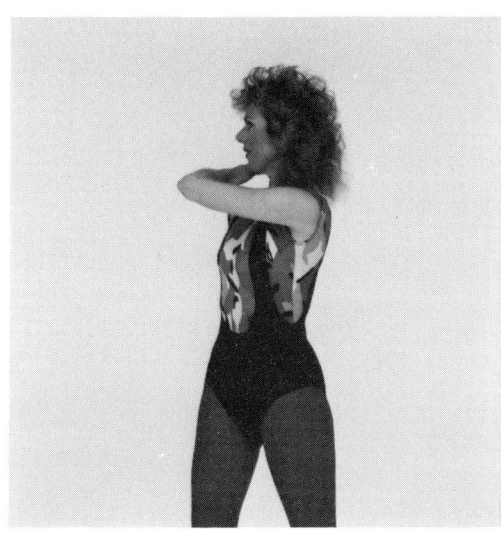 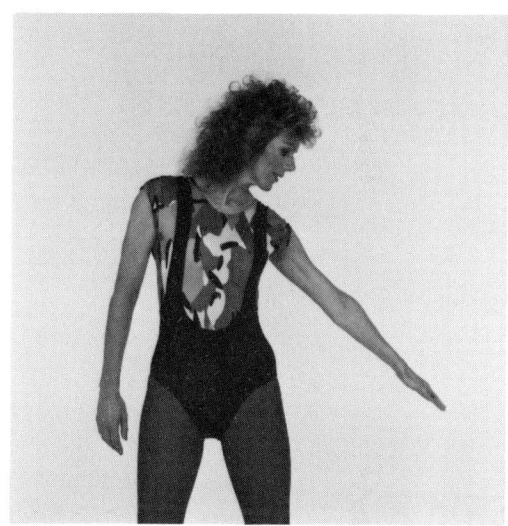

Bend your right arm and, guided by your elbow, circle your shoulder. Complete eight circles and repeat with your left arm.

Bend your right arm across your body at shoulder height and, as you do so, turn from your waist to look to your left. →

Swing your arm back down diagonally across your body. Continue flowing these two movements together, and repeat with your left arm.

THURSDAY: STAMINA DAY

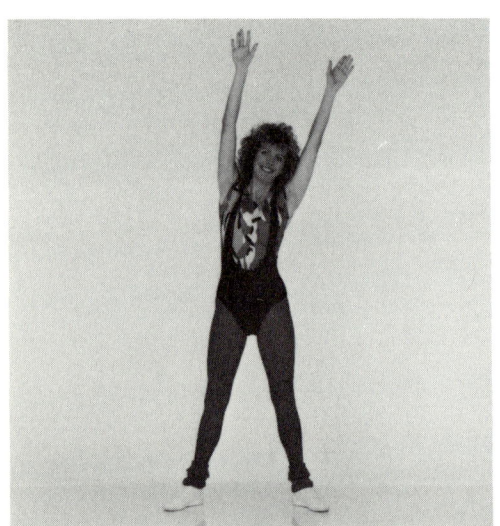

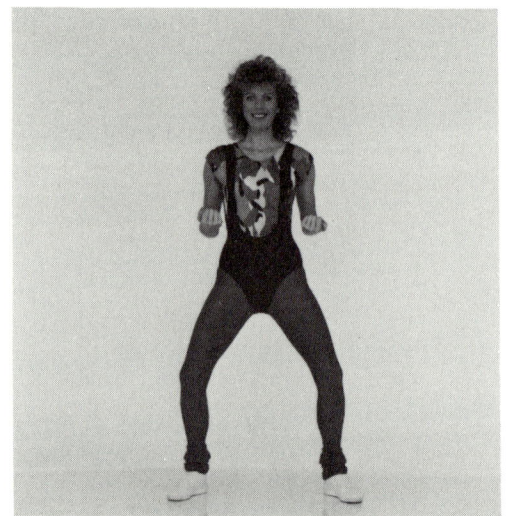

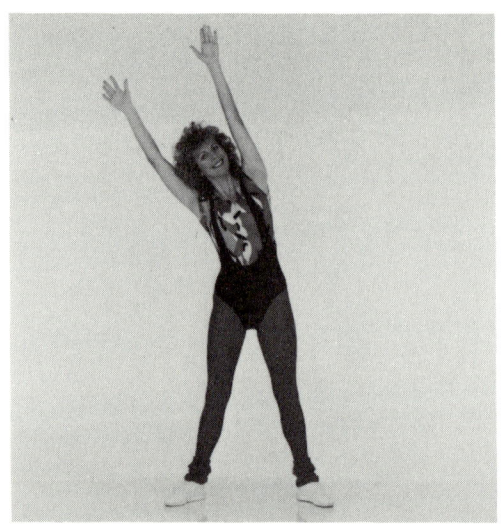

Raise both your arms up to your right diagonal. Stretch up out of your hips, tummy in, and reach just a little more to your right. →

Bend your legs as you bring both arms in, elbows tucked into the sides of the body. →

And stretch up with both arms, reaching for your left diagonal. Bend your legs again, drawing in both arms to your sides and keep flowing this exercise through these three movements.

THURSDAY: STAMINA DAY

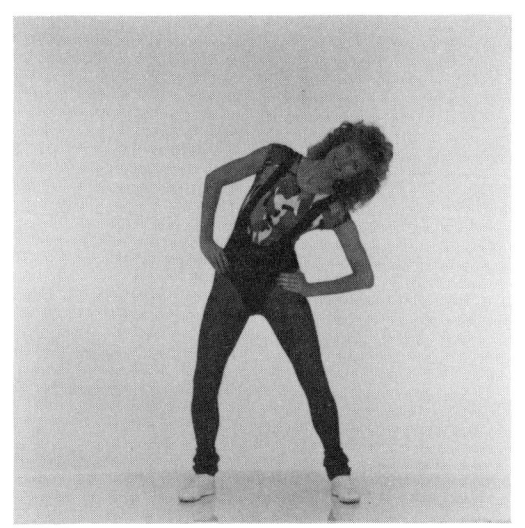 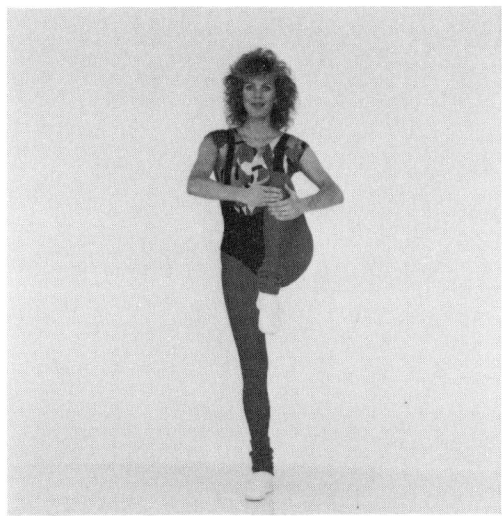 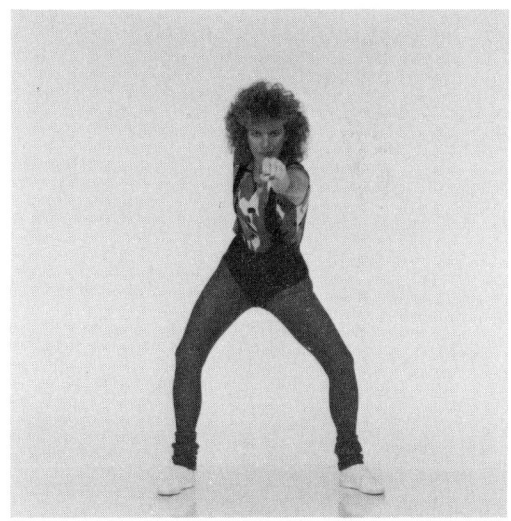

Bend your legs a little, place your hands at the top of your thighs and lean directly to your right side. Slowly centralize, and repeat the lean to your left side. Continue slowly stretching and working the waist in this way.

Raise your right knee and, lightly clasping it just below the knee with both hands, ease your leg up, helping to loosen both the leg and your right hip. Repeat the exercise with your left leg.

To complete your warm-up, think of all the things you would really like to hit — and punch through the air instead! Bend your legs and alternate punching out in front with each arm, using the strength of the shoulders. Hit hard, through to the fists.

THURSDAY: STAMINA DAY

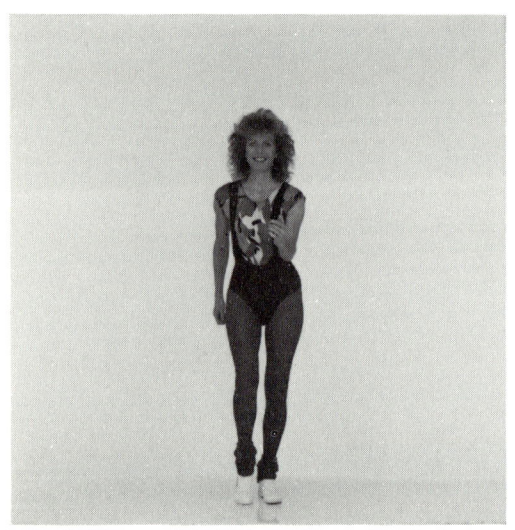 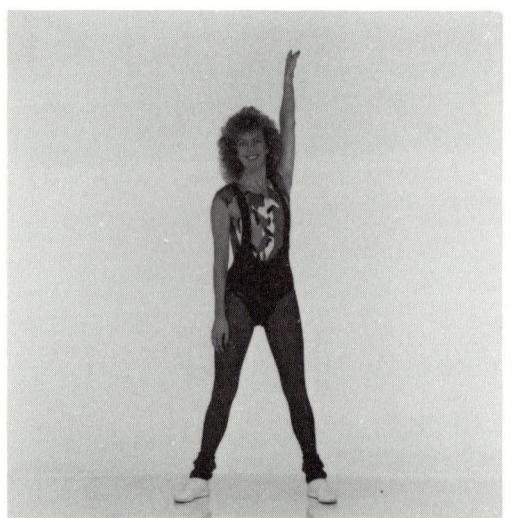 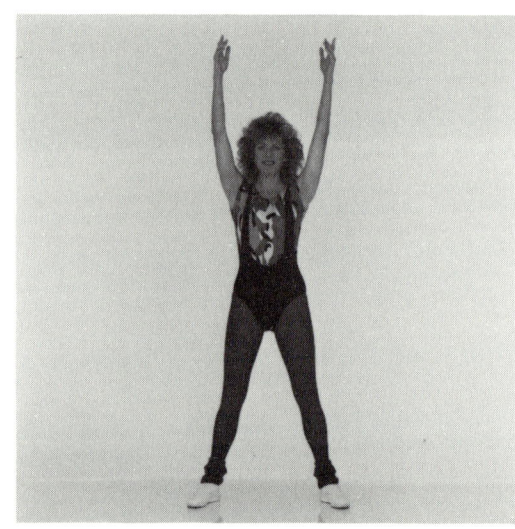

Lightly mark time on the spot, pushing through each foot and swinging each arm as if you were jogging — but without the running. Do this for about a minute.

With your feet and legs apart, circle your right arm forward and round, keeping your arm relaxed. Complete the circle eight times and repeat with your left arm.

Circle both arms together quite briskly. Feel your shoulders easing as you do so, but don't force your arms right behind you.

THURSDAY: STAMINA DAY

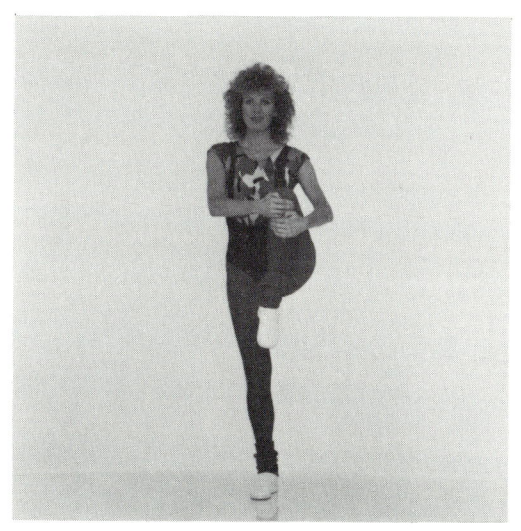 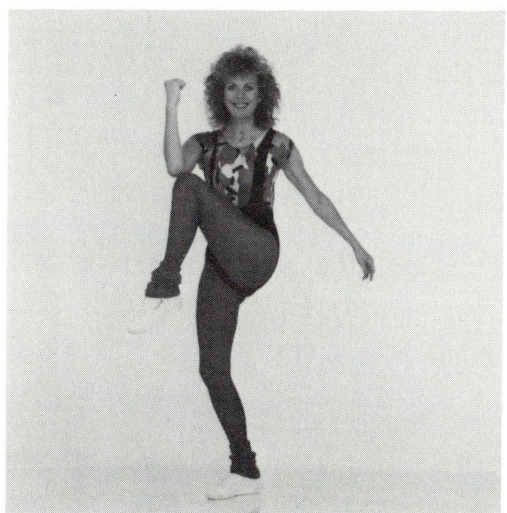 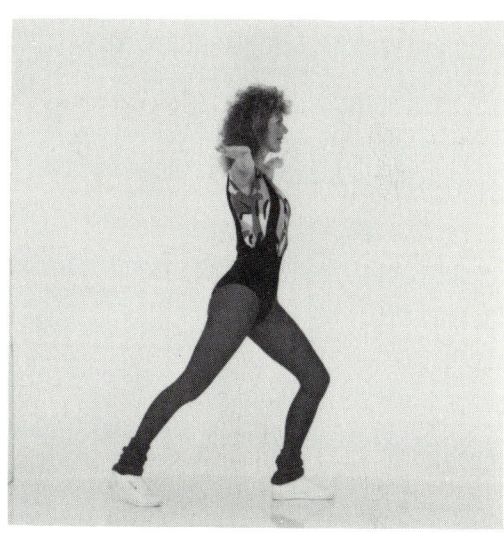

Stand straight. Raise your right knee, holding it just below the knee with both hands, and lower the leg. Repeat and change sides.

Raise your right leg, bending it across your body as high as you can. Swing your left elbow across your body at the same time, aiming to touch your knee. Lower your leg out to the side as you swing your elbow down to the side. Repeat and change sides.

Face your right side, arms outstretched at your sides, and stretch your left leg out behind you, bending your right knee and keeping your right foot flat on the floor. Hold that position, then repeat to your left.

THURSDAY: STAMINA DAY

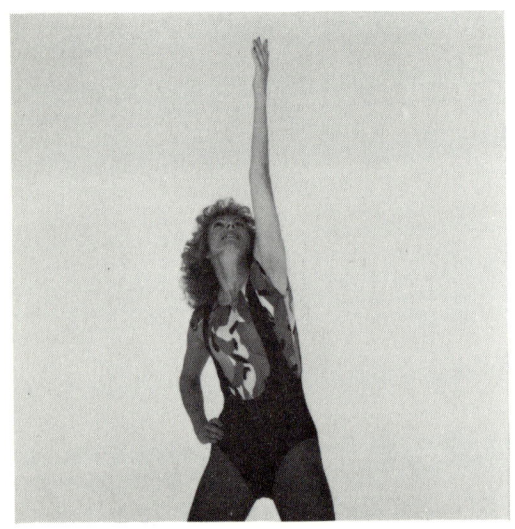

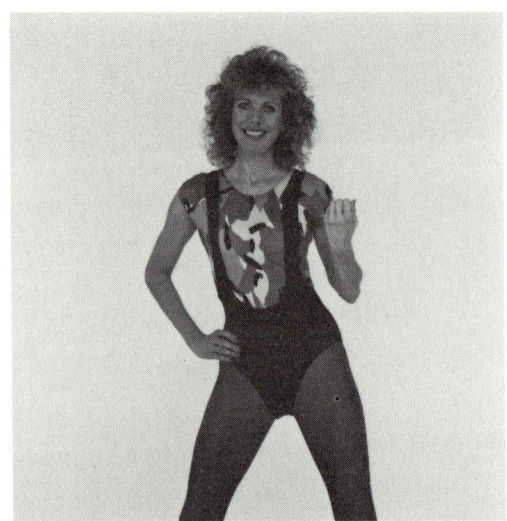

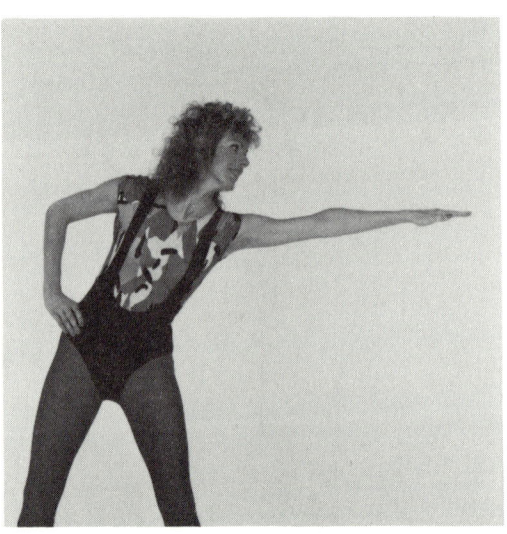

The following six movements are a sequence — each flowing into the next — to stretch your torso, trim your waist and help strengthen the back muscles. Place your left hand on your left hip and bend your legs. Reach up with your right arm and look up. →

Bend your right arm into your body, making a fist. →

Now reach out to your right side, leaning from your hips. →

THURSDAY: STAMINA DAY

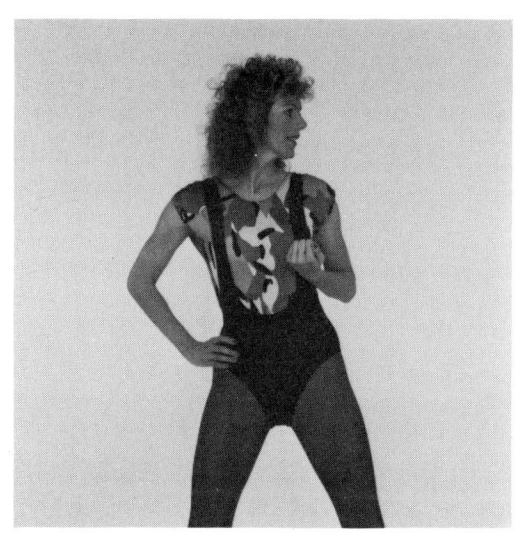 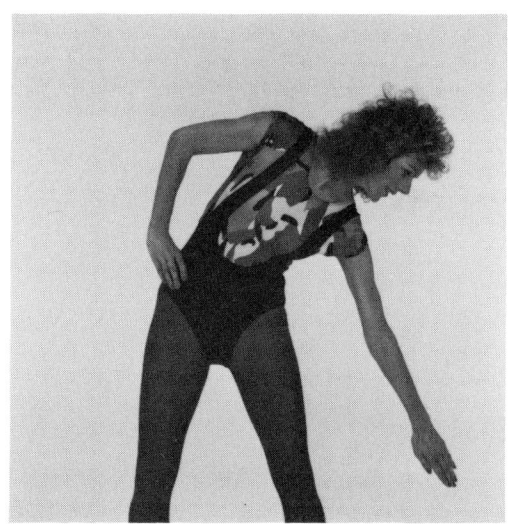 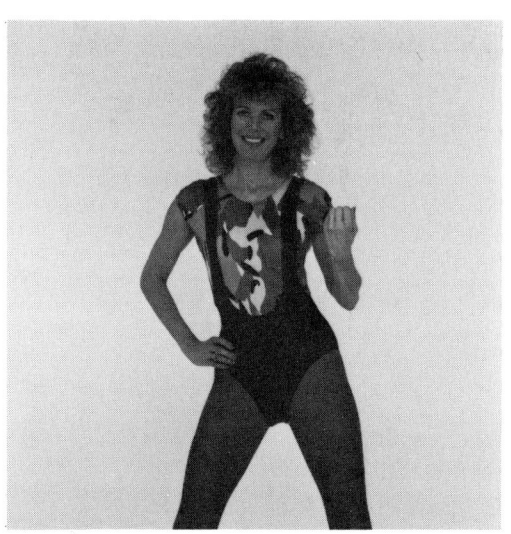

Bend your arm back into the side of your body, making a fist. →

Reach down, leaning over and looking down at your fingertips. →

Come up again, fist drawn in, and repeat the sequence. Change to your left.

75

THURSDAY: STAMINA DAY

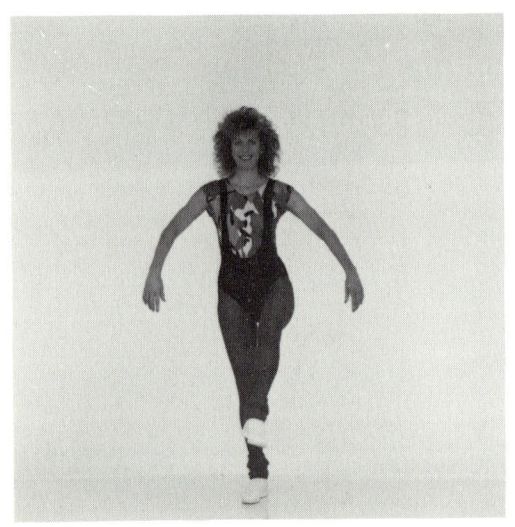

Loosely shake out the body. Make sure you are relaxed and warm.

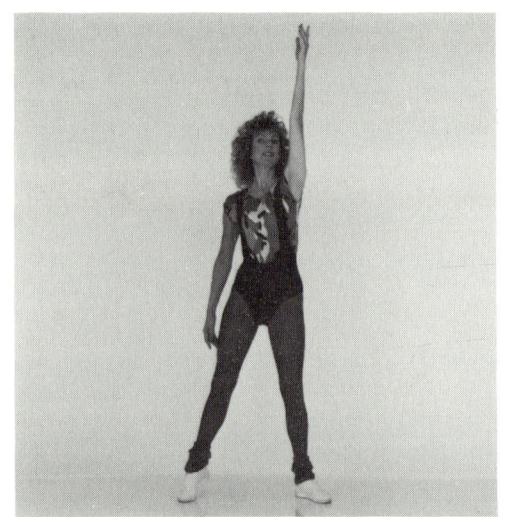

Stand with your legs and feet a comfortable distance apart, and raise your right arm and your left heel at the same time. Reach right up then lower your arm, making a fist at the side of your body, bend the elbow and lower the left heel. Continue to raise and lower arm and heel eight times and repeat on your left side.

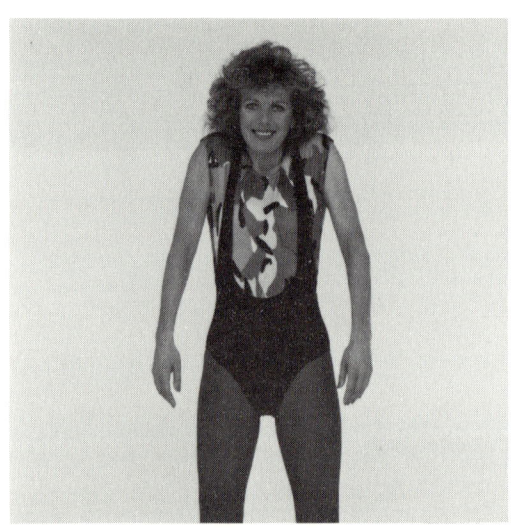

Loosely shrug both shoulders up towards your ears. Hold them there and lower them. Continue this movement up and down — as if saying 'I don't know!'

THURSDAY: STAMINA DAY

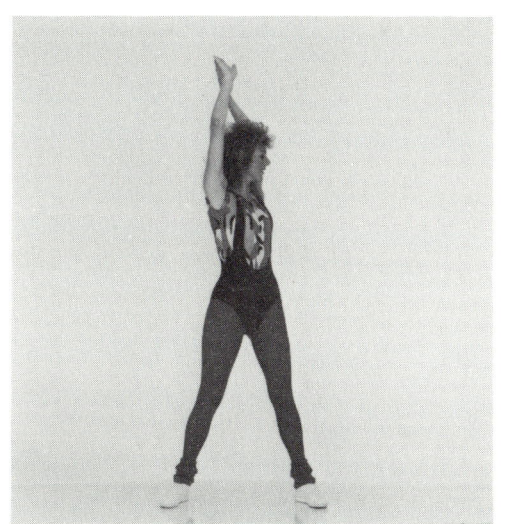

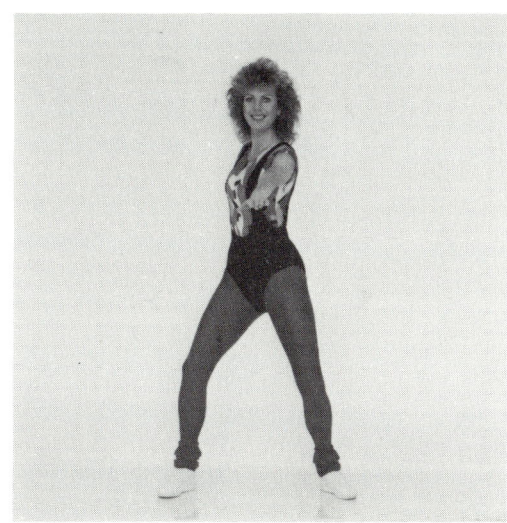

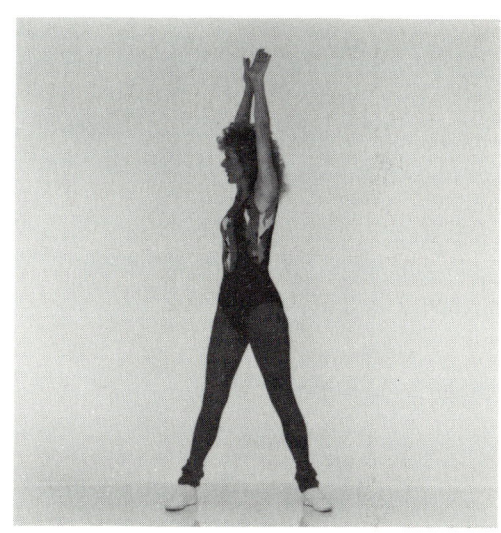

Turn from the waist to look to your right. As you do so, raise both arms out to the sides and up over your head. →

Lower them down by your sides as you bend the legs and face front to. →

Swing them up above your head while turning to face your left side. Lower them down again, face the front and bend your legs to continue the exercise flow.

THURSDAY: STAMINA DAY

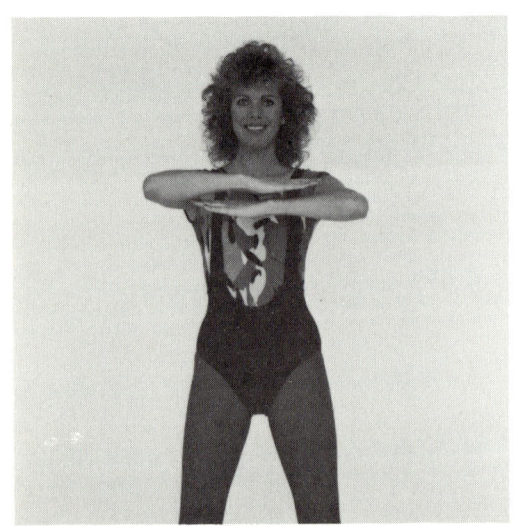 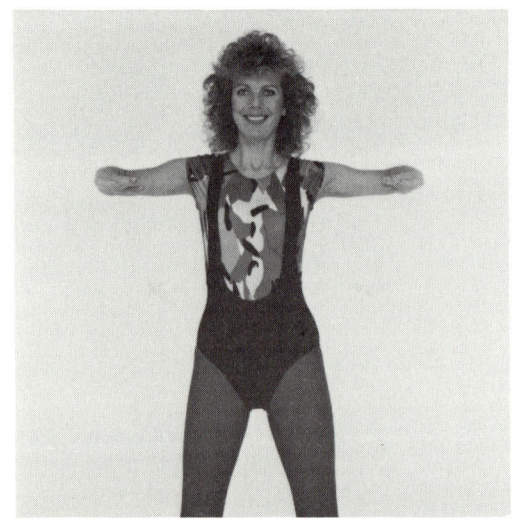 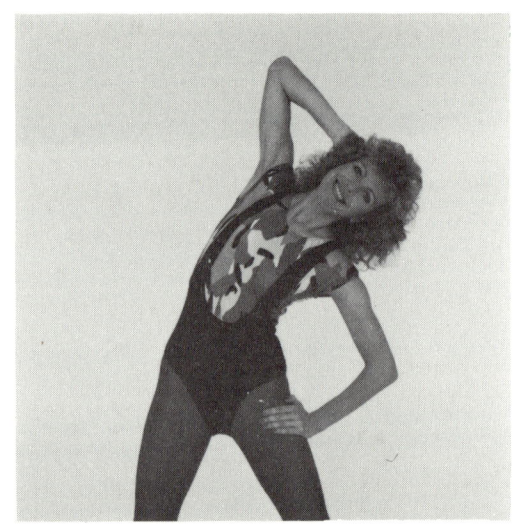

Raise both arms in front of you, bent at the elbows, chest height, one arm over the other — not touching. Keep your shoulders down.

Keeping your upper arms straight, ease your arms back — without any jerking movement. Feel the shoulder blades squeeze together behind you. Bring your arms back to the front.

Relax your knees. Place your right hand at the top of your right thigh and your left hand at the side of your head. Lean over to your right so that your left elbow is pointing towards the ceiling. Hold that position. Come up, change hands and lean to your left.

THURSDAY: STAMINA DAY

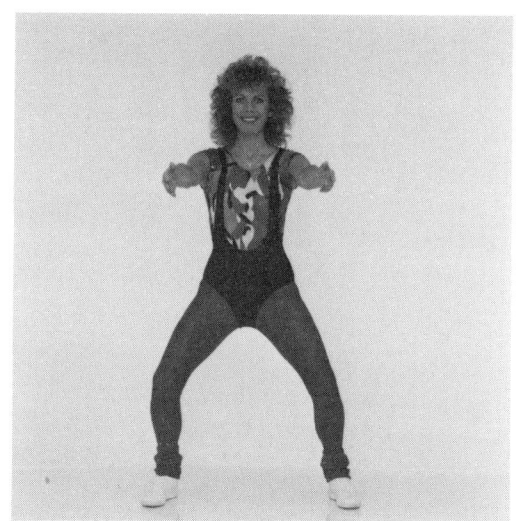

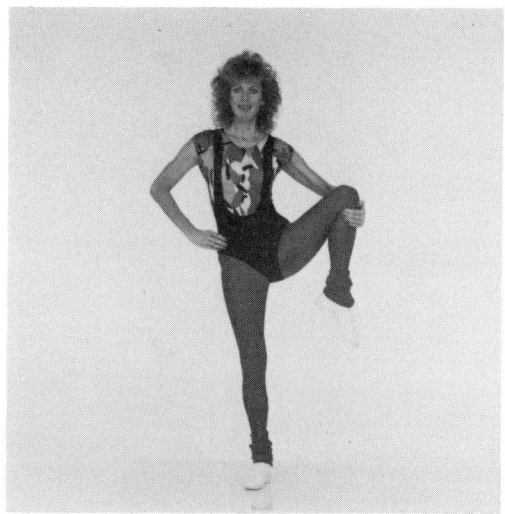

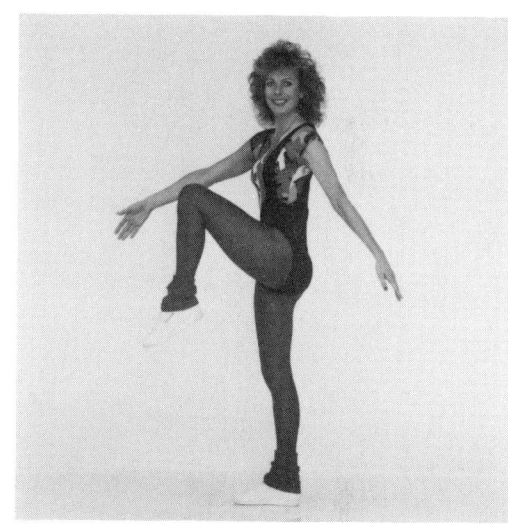

Standing with legs and feet apart, toes facing front, bend both legs, keeping the feet flat on the floor. Stretch both arms out in front and hold that position. Straighten your legs. You might only be able to do this three or four times to begin with.

Balance on your left leg and raise your right knee out to your right side — turning out from the very top of your leg. Hold it below the knee and try to ease the leg up, then lower your leg back down. Repeat with your left leg.

High march on the spot or around the room. Raise each knee as high as possible and swing your arms — feel those thighs working!

THURSDAY: STAMINA DAY

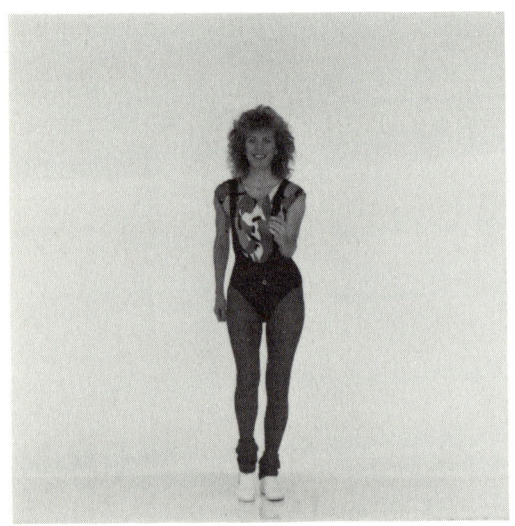

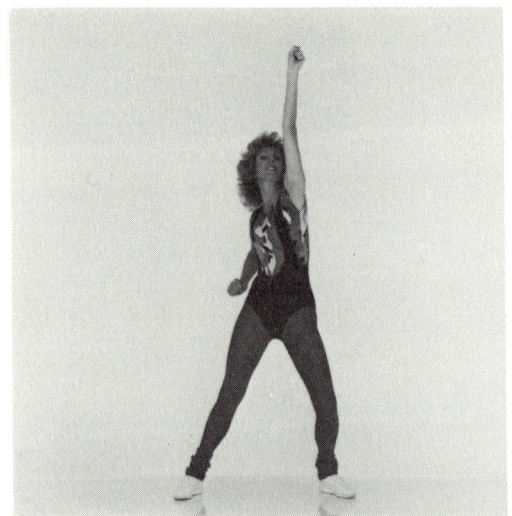

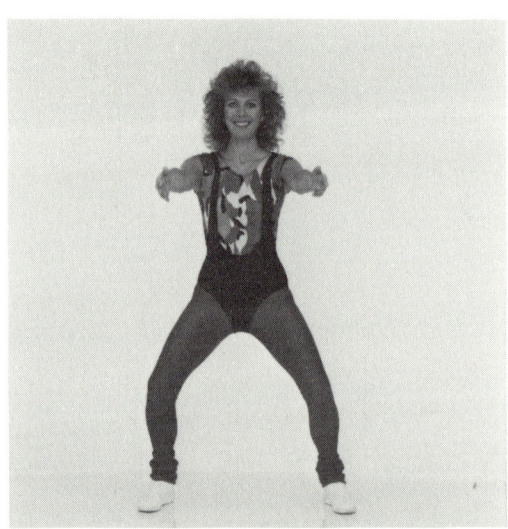

This is a 'miniature' version of marching. Lightly push through each foot, raising each a little off the ground, swinging the arms.

With your legs a comfortable distance apart, raise your right arm, hand in a fist, and bend your right leg. Lower your arm and repeat on the left side. You'll soon get into the swing of this exercise — the movements should flow together.

Bend both legs, feet flat on the floor, toes facing front, arms outstretched. Hold that position, straighten up and repeat.

THURSDAY: STAMINA DAY

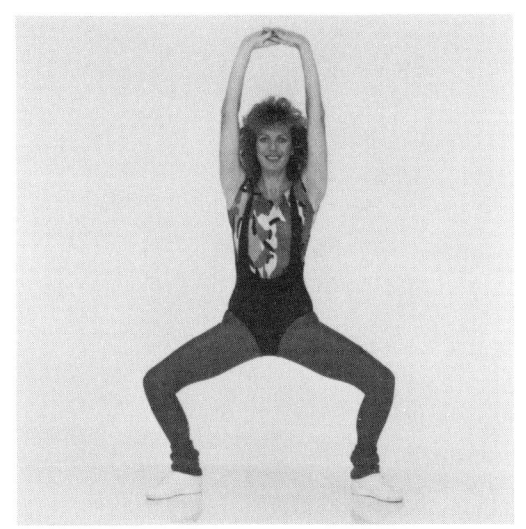 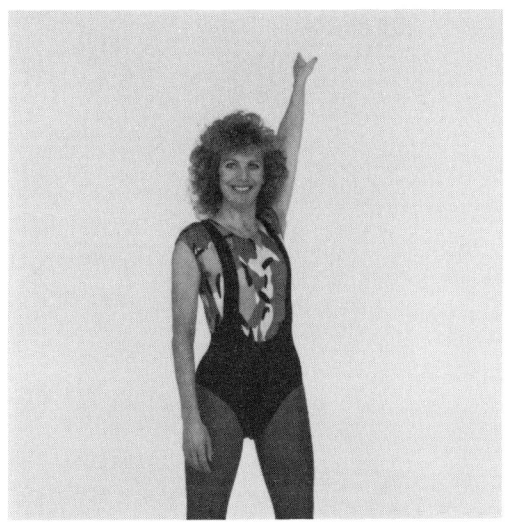 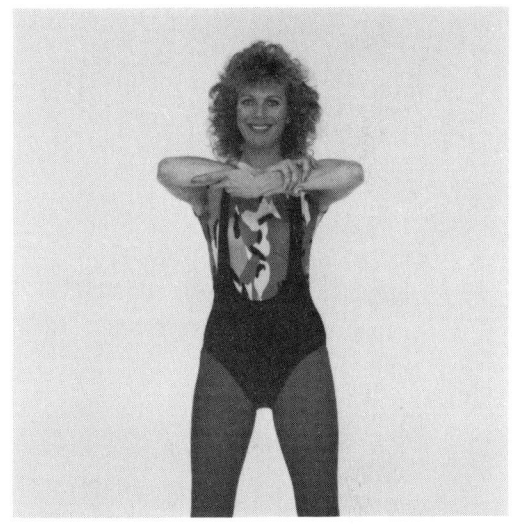

Turn the feet outwards so that the toes point out to their respective diagonals. Clasp your hands together, palms upward, and straighten your arms above your head. Bend your legs, tuck your bottom in and hold that position. Relax — then have another go!

Moving from the shoulder, circle your right arm forward and round in a continuous, flowing movement. Repeat with your left arm.

Bend your arms in front at chest height and hold each wrist with the opposite hand. Gripping the wrists, push those hands away from you. Feel those chest and boob muscles working!

THURSDAY: STAMINA DAY

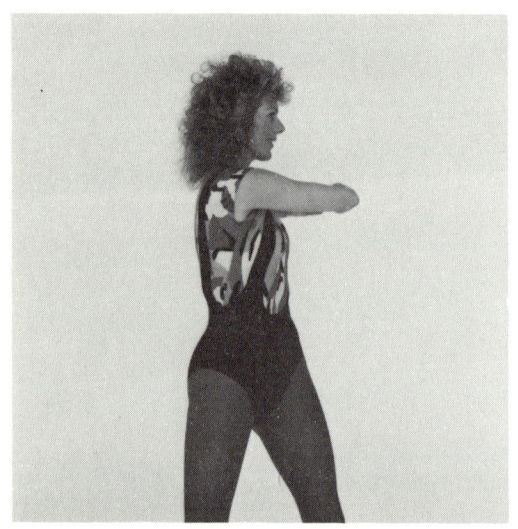

Still holding your wrists in front of you, turn from the waist as far round as you can go, and back to the front. Repeat and then turn to your left.

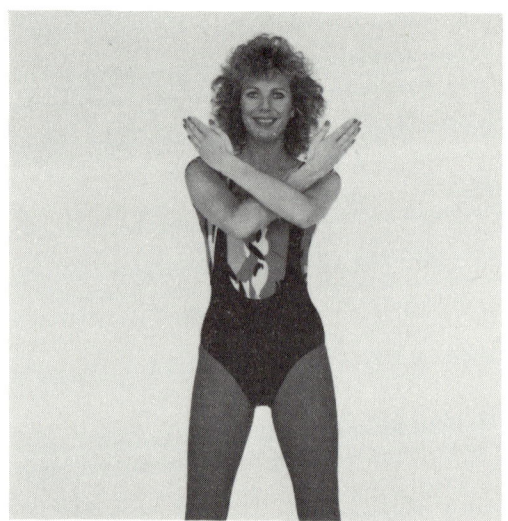

Start with your arms hanging loosely at your sides and swing them up in front of you so that they cross over at shoulder height. Repeat.

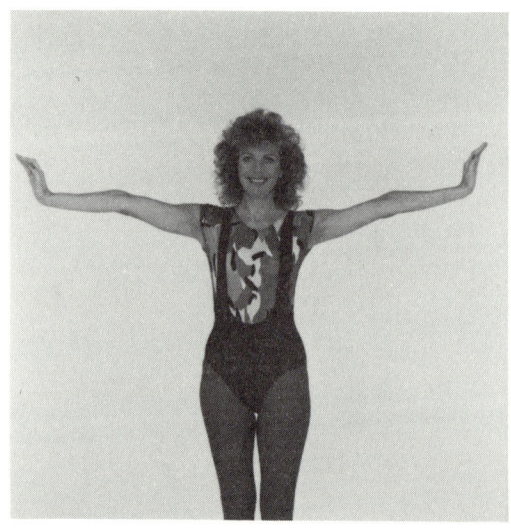

Stretch and straighten your arms out to the sides, fingers pointing to the ceiling. In large, slow circles, guide your arms and shoulders up and around — but keep those arms straight!

THURSDAY: STAMINA DAY

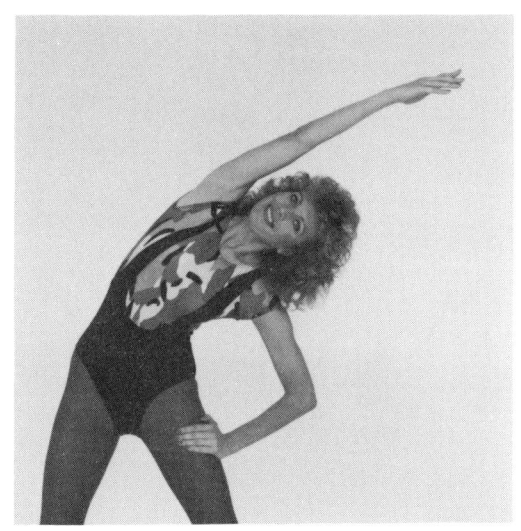
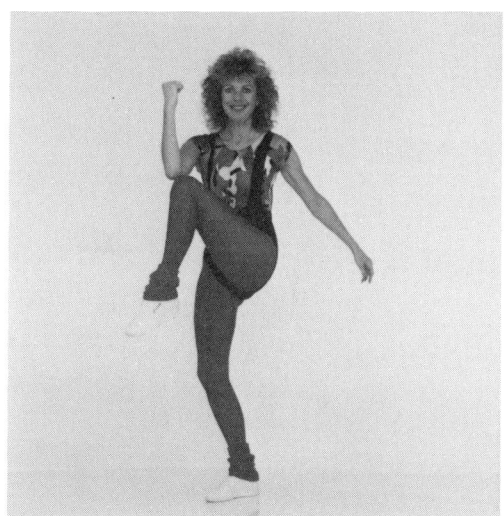
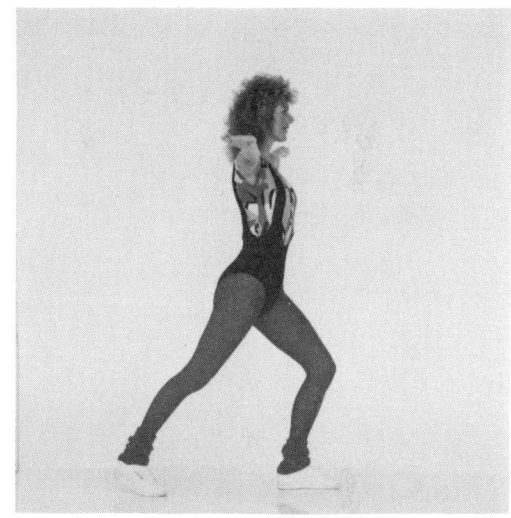

Bend your legs a little as you place your right hand at the top of your thigh. Raise your left arm and curve it over your head, reaching over as far as you can. Enjoy the stretch. Change arms and stretch over to your left.

Raise your right knee across your body and aim to touch it with your left elbow. Don't lean — keep upright. Lower the leg and repeat as many times as you can before changing legs.

Lunge to your right side, bending your right leg, foot flat on the floor, and extending your left leg behind you, arms outstretched at the side for balance. Hold this position, then turn to face your left and repeat.

Friday

> **WARM UP** Today the warm-up exercises are on the floor — variety is the spice of life! As before, do each exercise eight times, or as many as you can achieve.

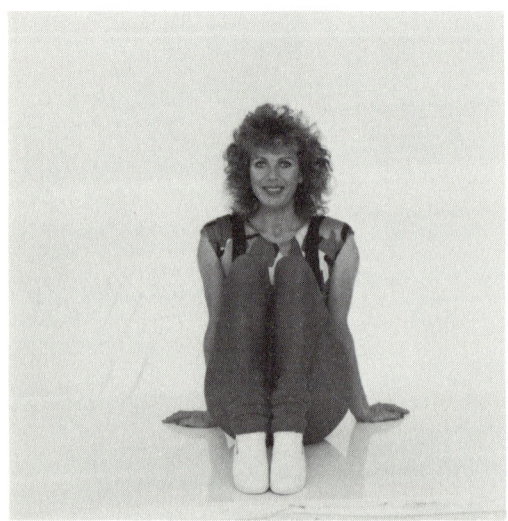

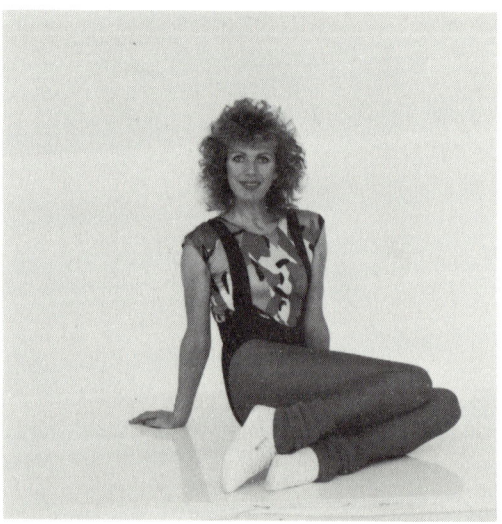

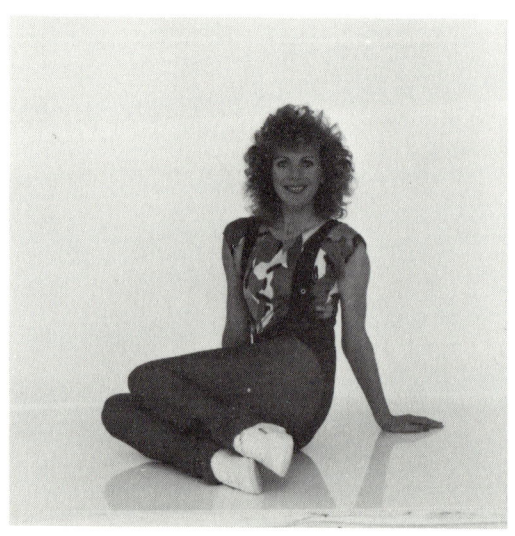

Sit on the floor, hands on the floor either side. Draw your knees up, toes pointing on the floor. Sit up. →

Keeping your legs together, let both knees roll across your body so that your right knee comes down to touch the floor. Try to keep your torso facing front so that you are working from the waist. Bring both legs back to the centre. →

And repeat to your left.

FRIDAY: WARM UP

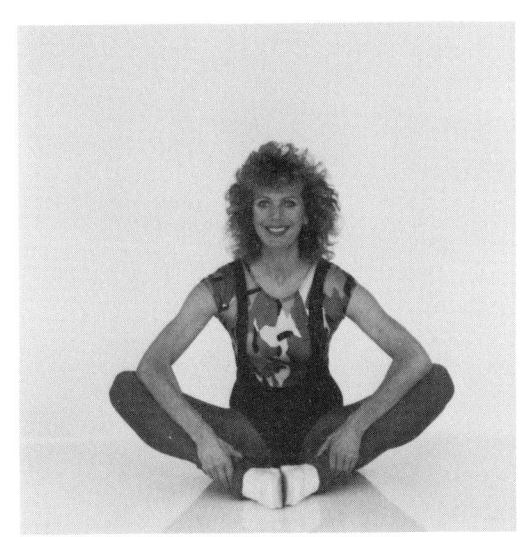 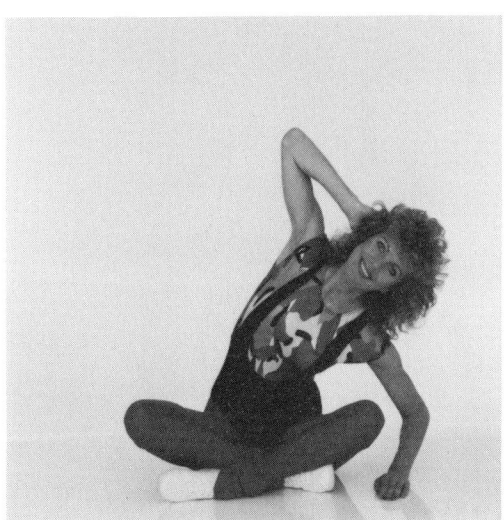 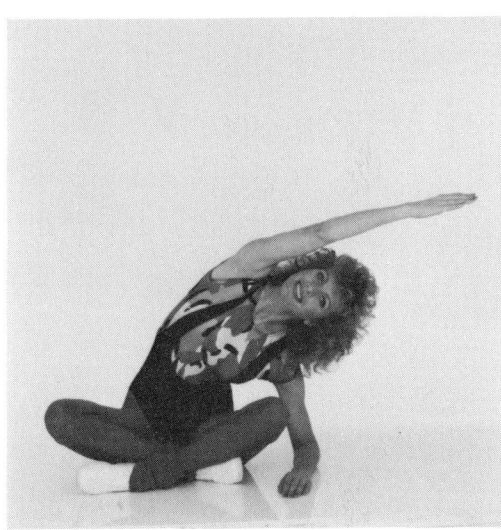

Sit with your knees flopping out, soles of the feet touching. Grasp both ankles and, with the help of your hands, practise correct posture by 'sitting tall' and then collapsing into the centre.

Sitting cross-legged, place your right hand on the floor, bend your left arm and rest the fingers lightly on the side of your head and lean to your right side. Keep your left elbow pointing upwards and gently reach over eight times. Change arms and lean to your left.

This time curve your whole arm over your head and lower on to your right forearm. Change arms and stretch over with your right arm.

FRIDAY: WARM UP

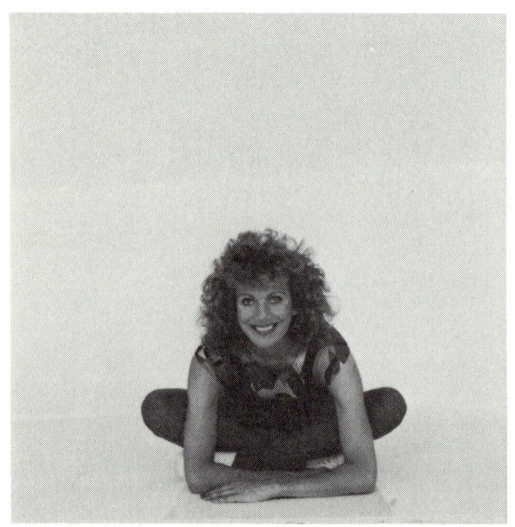 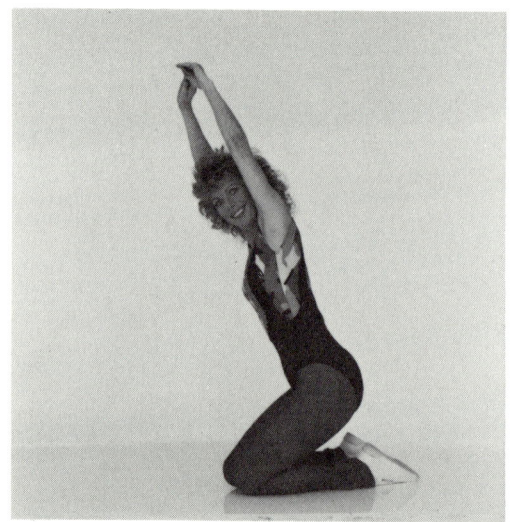 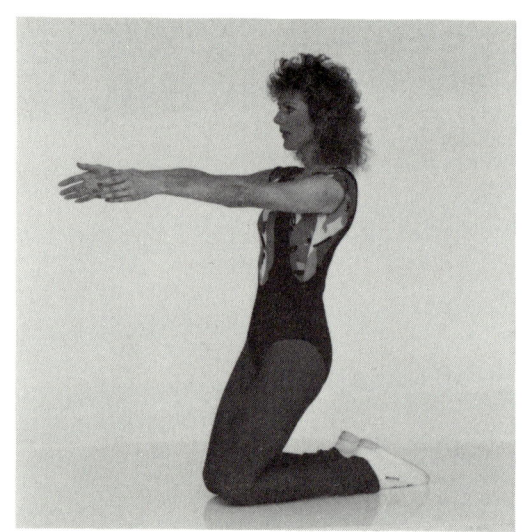

You might not be able to do this fully, but see how far you can lean forward. Sitting cross-legged, place your hands on the floor in front of you. Gently flatten your back as you lower yourself on to your forearms — *don't* over-stretch.

Kneel down and clasp your hands above your head. Raise your bottom so that you are not sitting on your feet. Circle the hips and bottom by sinking round to the right — just above the feet — and coming up again round to the left. Repeat, circling the other way.

Kneeling upright, arms outstretched in front, slowly lean back — don't do a back bend — *lean* the torso back, keeping the back straight. Feel the stretch on the thighs, and slowly come forward again.

FRIDAY: WARM UP

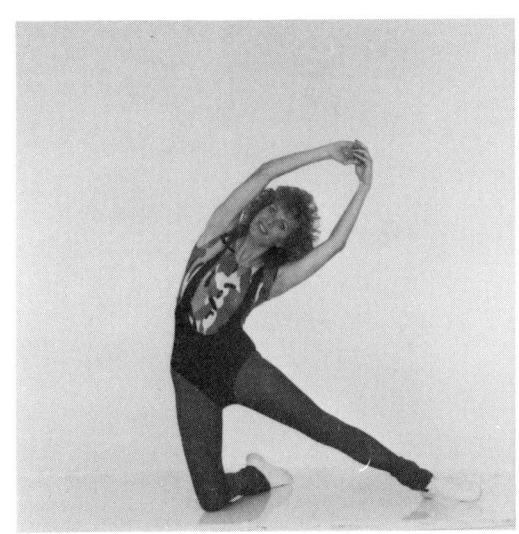
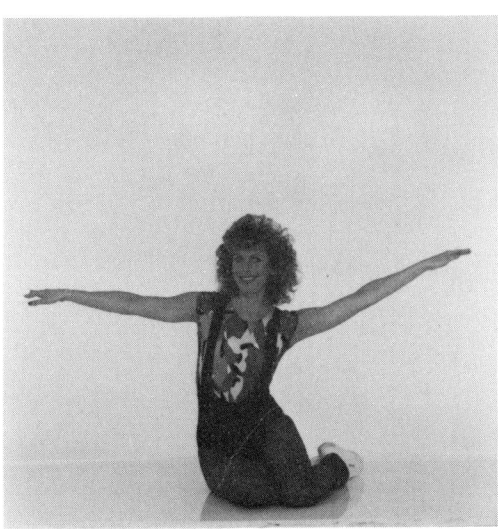
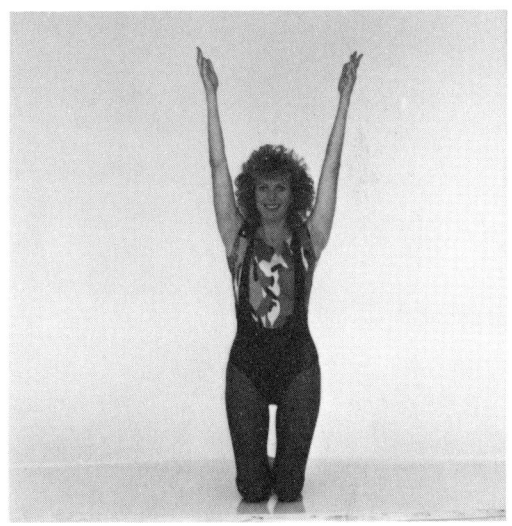

Kneel on your left leg and extend your right leg to the side. Holding your hands above your head, lean to the right. With a tiny movement reach over eight times. Change legs and lean to your left.

Sit with both legs bent and tucked under your right side, arms stretched out either side. Lean towards your right. →

Now try swooping your arms forward and up as you push up through your thighs on to your knees. This action is one single movement and you might not achieve it to begin with, your thighs need to be strong and your balance and coordination good. Come down from the kneeling position with both legs bent and tucked under your left side. Lean to your left and repeat.

FRIDAY: POP DANCE

POP DANCE

A great way to exercise! Let's get 'on the move' and 'in the mood' for the weekend! These exercises will keep you in rhythm with your body, so choose an up-tempo record and coordinate to the music.

Each movement should be 'big': if you are stepping to the side, make it a big step; if you're clapping your hands together, make it flamboyant — you could even try making up your own sequences.

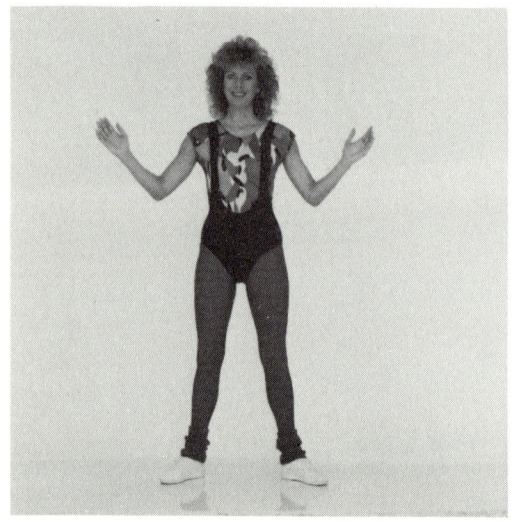

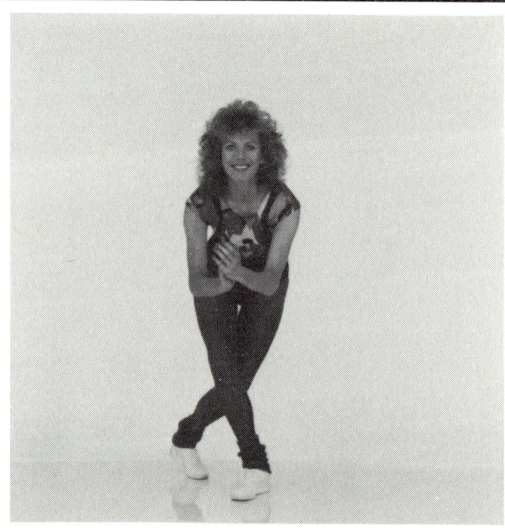

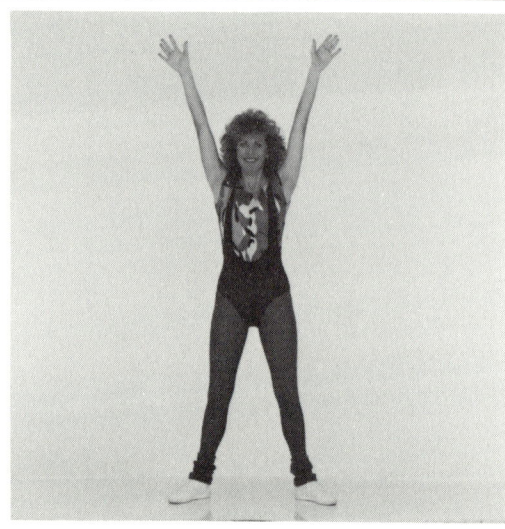

Master these first four steps — if you find them hard to follow, practise the footwork first.

Stand with your feet and legs a comfortable distance apart and your arms open. →

Bend your left leg as you cross your right foot behind it, heel raised. At the same time, clap your hands and crouch forward, head up. →

Stand tall, stretching both arms above your head and step on your right foot. →

FRIDAY: POP DANCE

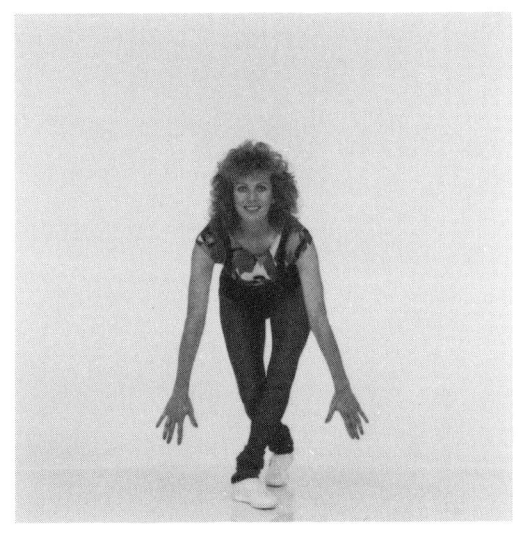 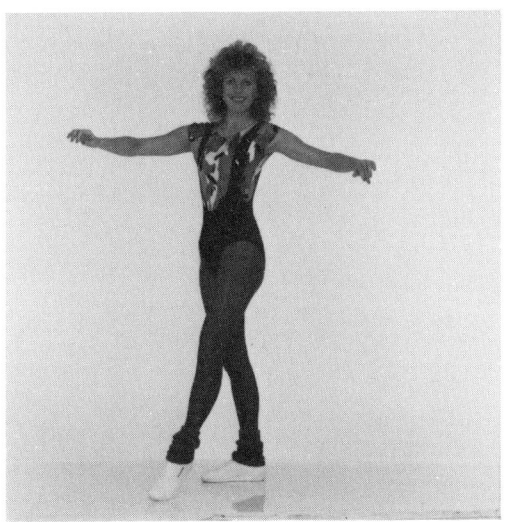 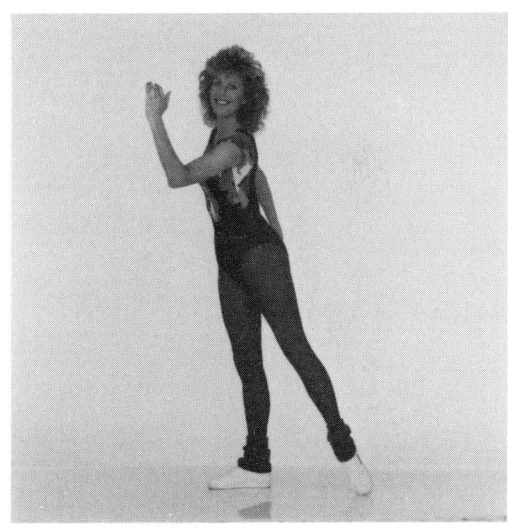

Cross your left foot behind your right, bend both legs and shoot your arms down either side of your body. Keep repeating this sequence.

Turn your body to your left diagonal as you move your right foot in front across your body, toes touching the floor, swing your left arm in front. →

Point your right foot behind, swinging your right arm up in front. Do these two steps four times and repeat using your left leg.

FRIDAY: POP DANCE

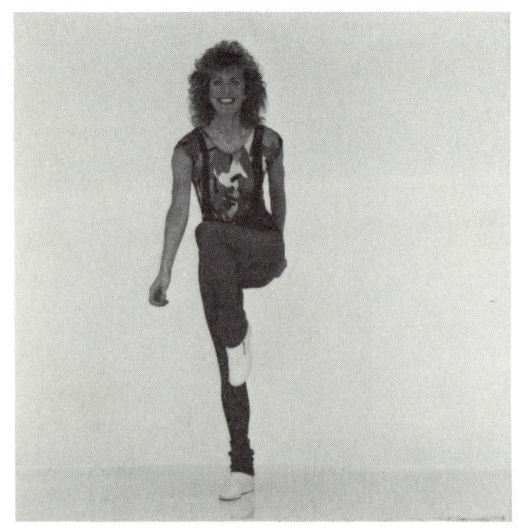
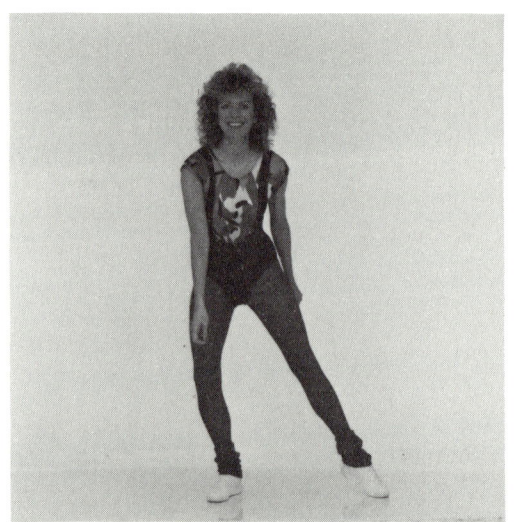
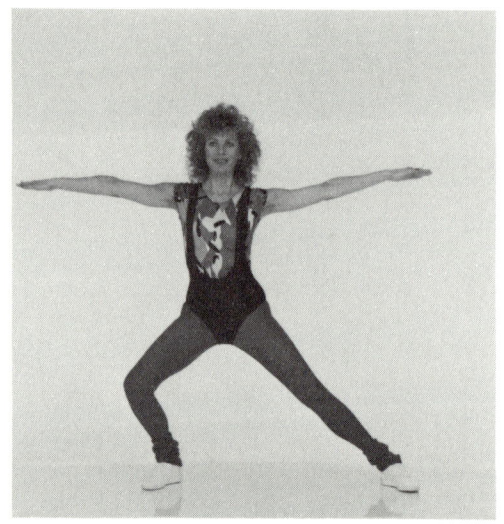

On the next beat quickly face your left diagonal again and jump your right knee up across your body. →

And land lightly, touching the floor with your right foot to the side. Repeat these two movements together four times and then continue, facing your right diagonal, working your left leg.

Slow the pace down by lunging from side to side. Step your left leg to the side and bend it, extending both arms out to your sides. Hold for one beat, then transfer your weight by bending your right leg. Repeat four times each side, holding for one beat between the changes. Now try it in double-time: do eight fast changes, clapping as you change the lunge.

FRIDAY: POP DANCE

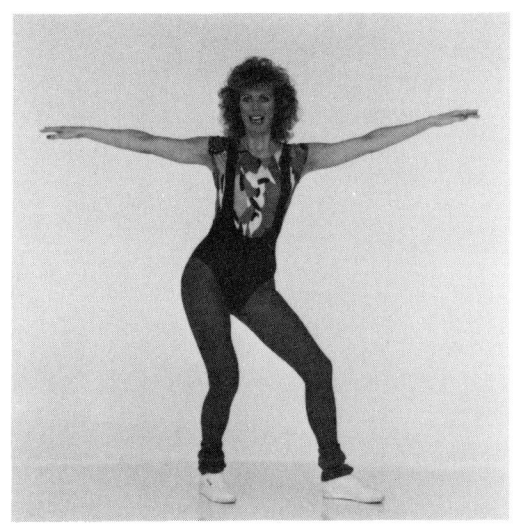 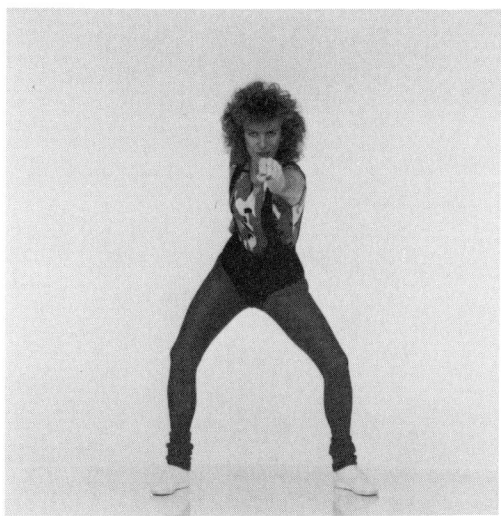 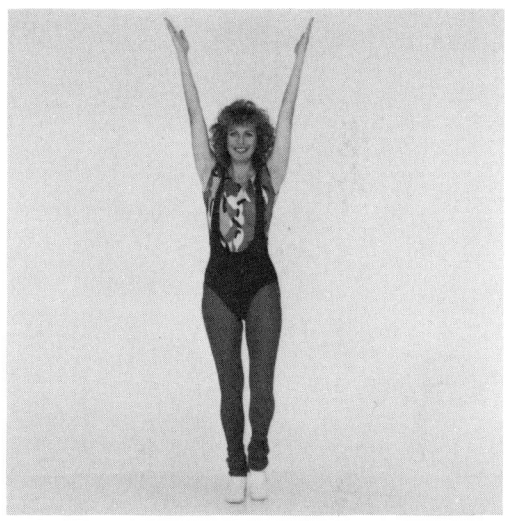

Swing those hips in time for your Saturday night parties! Bend both legs and try to do whole circles, guiding your hips round to your left, front, right and behind. Then try swinging them from side to side.

With your feet apart and your legs bent, pretend to shadow-box with a partner. Punch straight in front, through the air, and then do double punches. You can also do this exercise punching straight above your head and alternating each arm — but only single punches.

To finish off, get on the move again. Lightly marking time with a tiny jogging movement, raise both arms above your head, open them wide and clap your hands sixteen times.

Go on — improvise!

FRIDAY: LEG EXERCISES STAGE I

LEG EXERCISES STAGE I

It takes time to build up muscle strength, particularly in the thighs. Any trembling of the muscles means they have been pushed to their limits, so do not continue — leave this exercise until you come round to it again next week. Also, do not overshoot the gap when you exercise with your legs apart — it's tempting, but you have to learn to walk before you can run, so take your time.

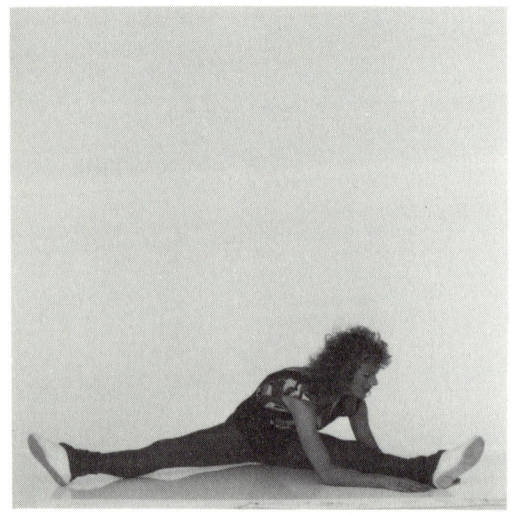
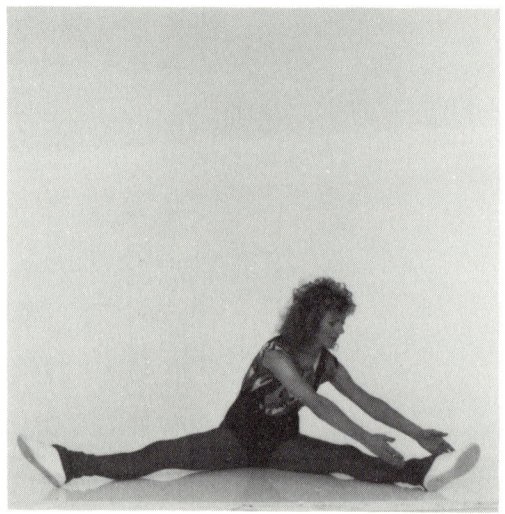
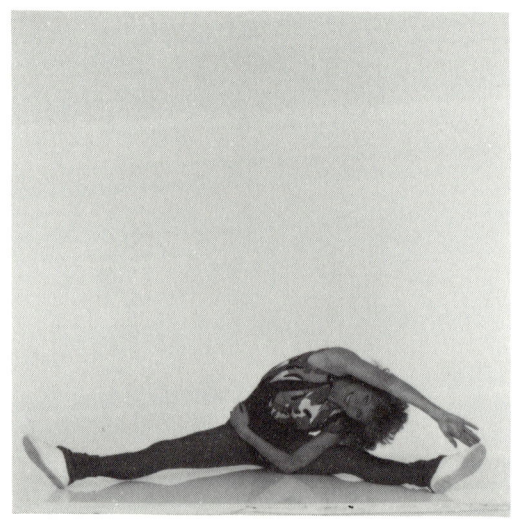

Sit on the floor, legs apart and, turning from the waist, lean your torso directly in line with your right leg. Try not to hunch your back. With a tiny movement, reach forward towards your toes. Change sides and try to your left.

Now try reaching for your toes with both hands, keeping your back straight, tummy in, and hold the stretch. Change sides.

Sit up and raise your left arm over your head, bending your right arm over your body so that it almost touches your left hip. Turn from the waist and reach over with your left arm, aiming to touch your right foot with your left fingers — one day!

FRIDAY: LEG EXERCISES STAGE I

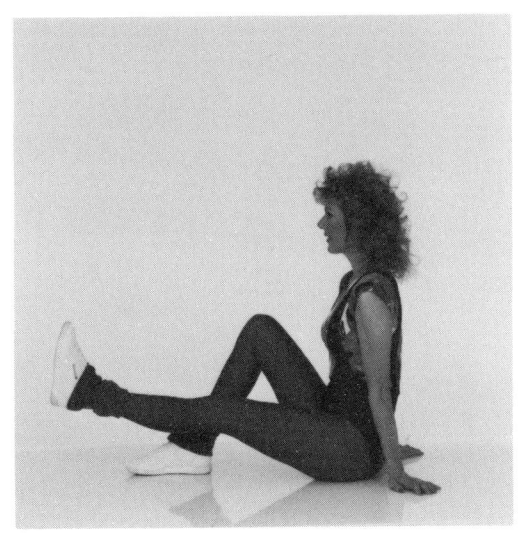
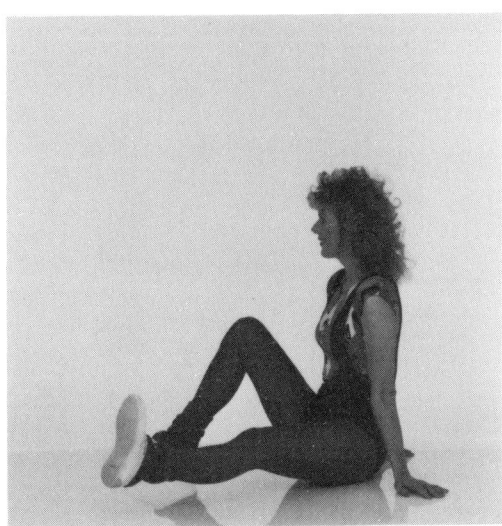
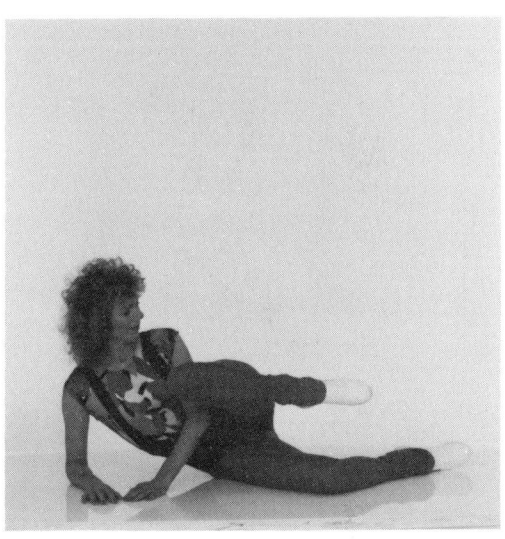

Sit up and place both hands behind you to support your weight. Bend your right leg and keep the foot flat on the floor. Keep your left leg straight out in front, toes pointing to the ceiling, and raise and lower it — keeping it off the floor. Change legs.

From the same starting position as the previous exercise, raise your left leg, open it out to your side and 'swing' it shut. Open and close your leg, keeping it off the floor. Change legs.

Lie on your left side, bending your left arm and leg underneath you. Raise and bend your right leg up towards your chest. →

FRIDAY: LEG EXERCISES STAGE I

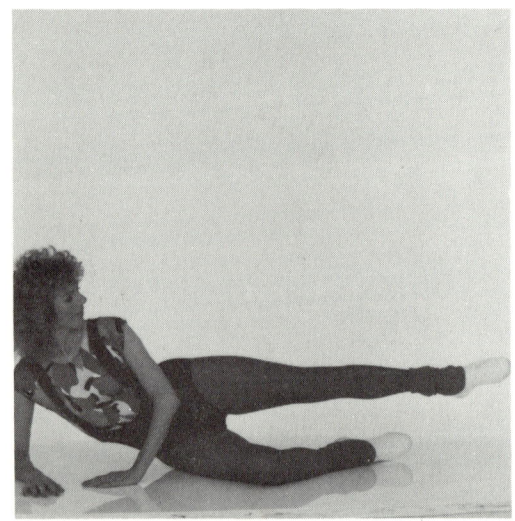

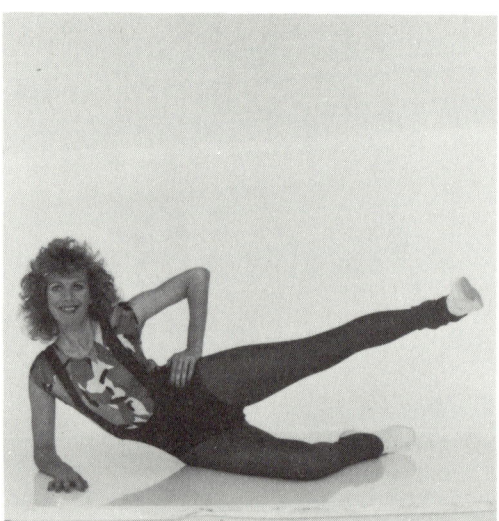

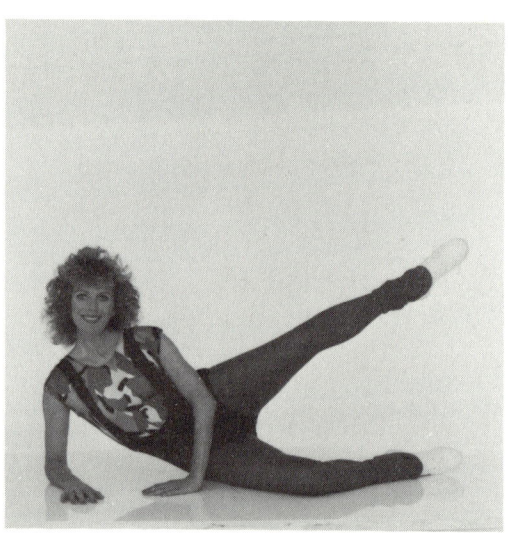

Extend your right leg away from you, off the ground. →

Raise and lower your right leg, keeping the foot flat, toes pointing to the front. Keep the foot off the floor as you lower it. →

Bend your right leg and raise and lower it slowly, this time with the toes pointing straight. Now change sides and repeat these four movements, working your left leg.

FRIDAY: LEG EXERCISES STAGE I

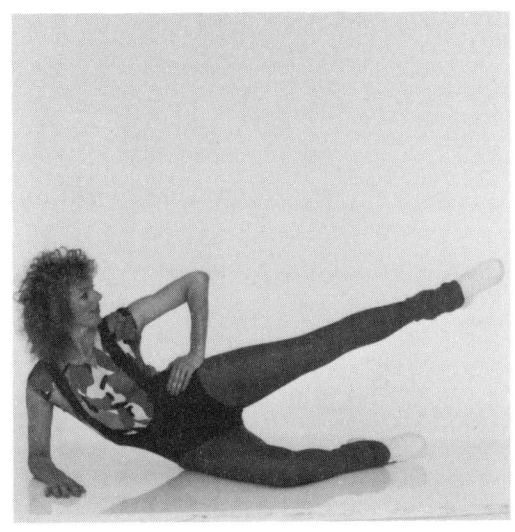

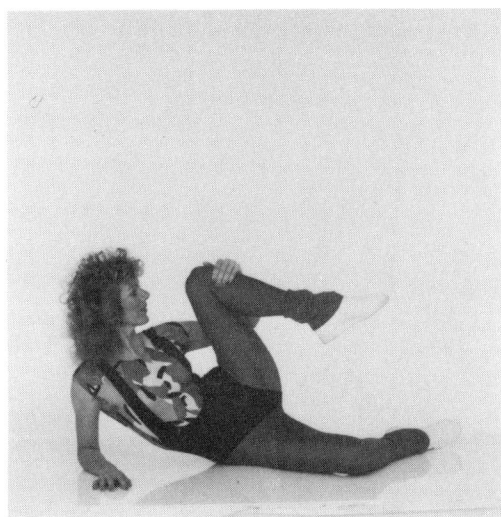

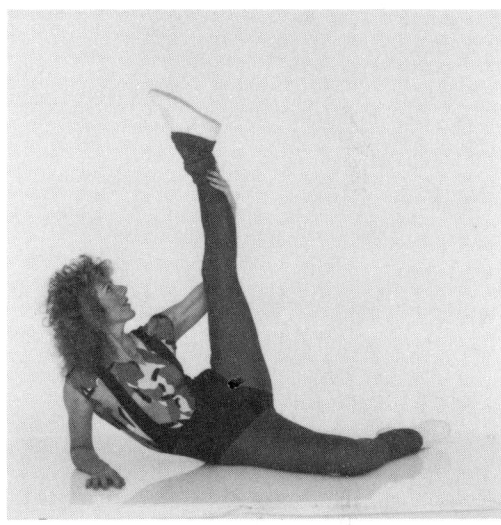

Lie back on your left side, raise your right leg and circle the leg slowly forward and round. 'Draw' large circles in the air. →

Bend your right knee in so that it points towards your head, and hold it lightly below the kneecap. →

Straighten the leg down, then kick straight up in the air, turning out from the very top of the leg. Catch it below the calf. Repeat these three movements and change sides.

FRIDAY: TUMMY STAGE II

TUMMY STAGE II

Here we go. Achieve and progress, but don't push it. Even people — men and women — who have been exercising regularly for years can't achieve all these exercises. Do what you can at first, and build up the number week by week. Don't forget to chart your progress.

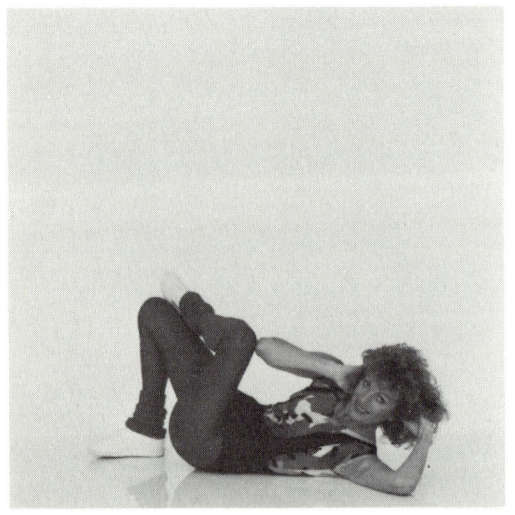

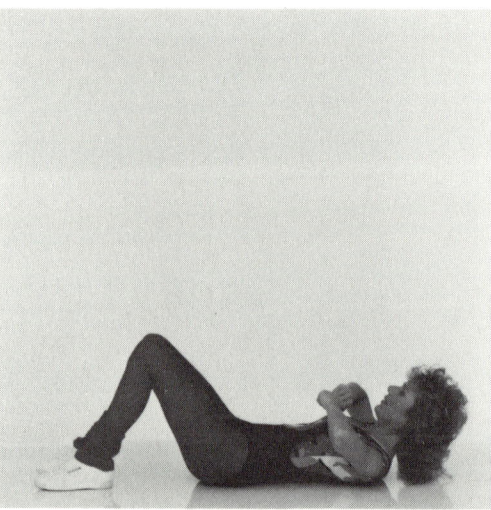

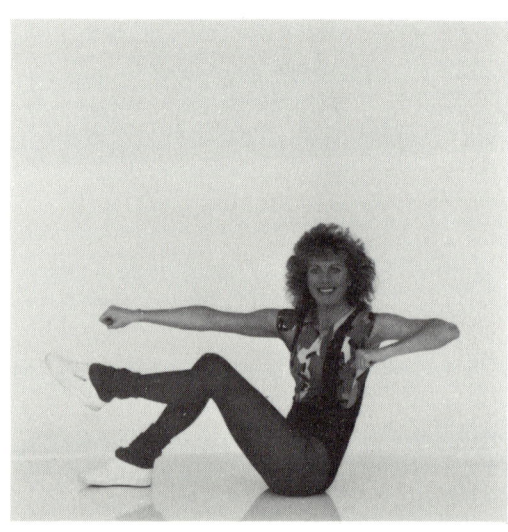

Bend your right leg and keep the foot flat on the floor. Cross your left leg over so that the side of the left foot rests above the right knee. Sit up to touch your left knee with your right elbow. Sit up and lie back in rhythm, keeping your head off the floor. How many can you do before changing sides?

This is a difficult one to achieve — I call it the 'archery' tummy exercise, because of the use of the arms. Lie flat on your back, draw your knees up. Raise your head off the ground and never let it go back any further than illustrated. Bend your arms in front, at chest height. →

In one move, sit up through a curved spine, using the tummy muscles. As you raise your right leg pull your left arm back, as if pulling back an arrow. Turn to see your left side. Lie back and repeat using your right side.

FRIDAY: TUMMY STAGE II

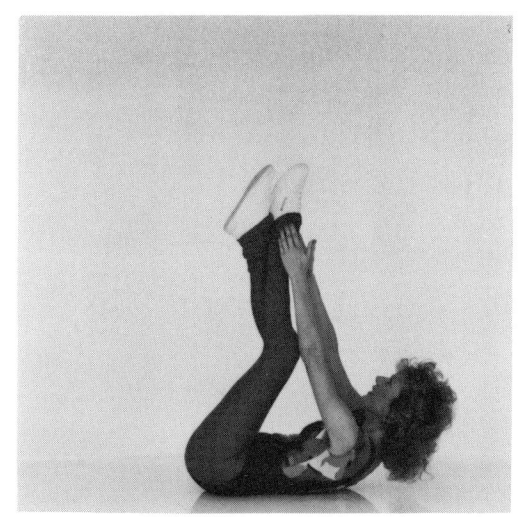

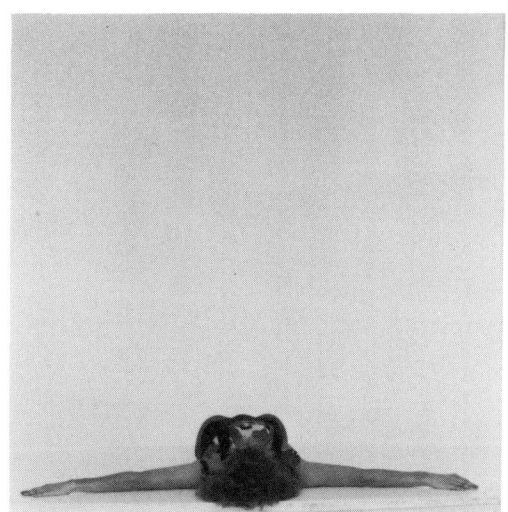

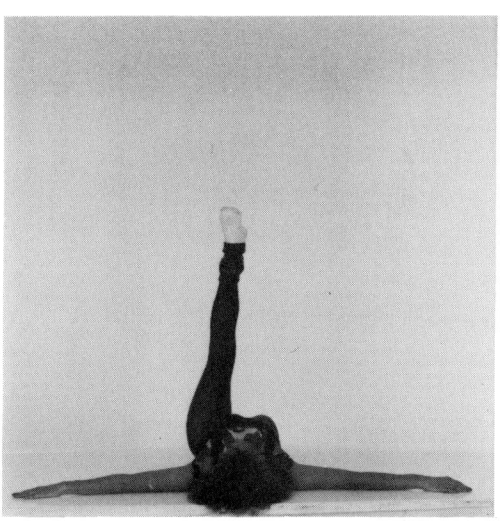

Raise both legs in the air, locking the feet by crossing the legs at the ankles. Keeping your head off the floor, reach up off your shoulders for your ankles. Repeat. Don't forget to fill in your progress chart with this exercise.

The next six movements are a sequence — easy to follow and highly effective. You should study them carefully before having a go.

Lie flat on your back, arms outstretched to your sides. →

Raise your left leg straight in the air. →

FRIDAY: TUMMY STAGE II

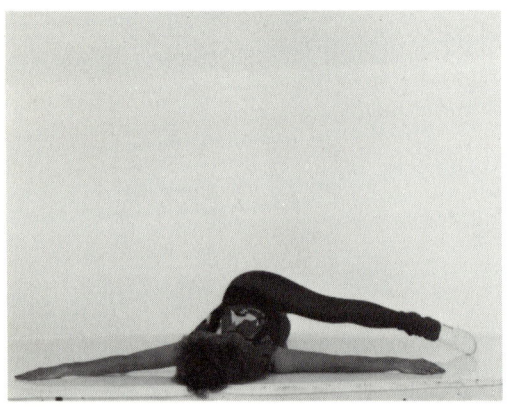

Guide it over to your right side, towards your right hand. As you do so, turn your head away to the left. →

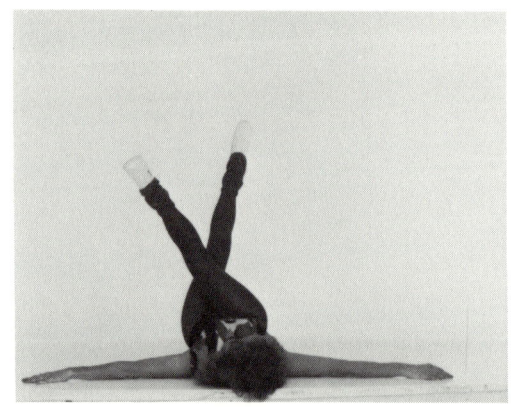

As you raise your leg back up to the centre, bring your right leg straight up to cross over in front of your left leg, as it goes down to the floor. →

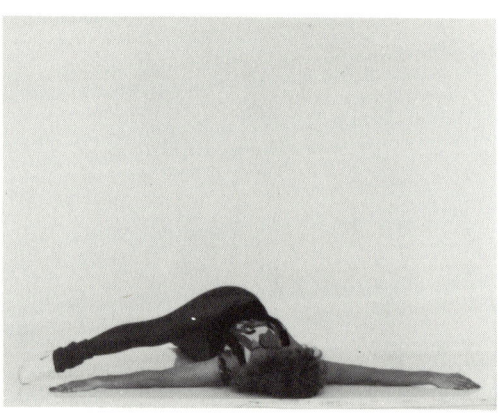

Take your right leg over towards your left hand and turn your head to your right. →

FRIDAY: TUMMY STAGE II

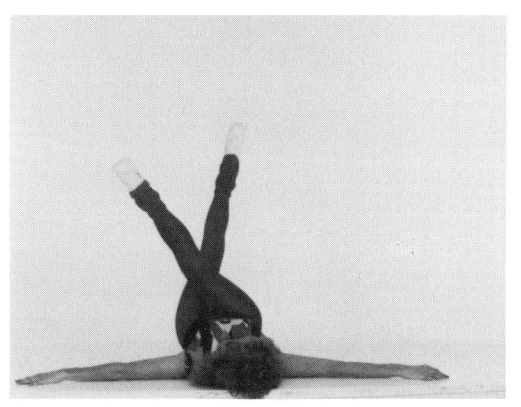 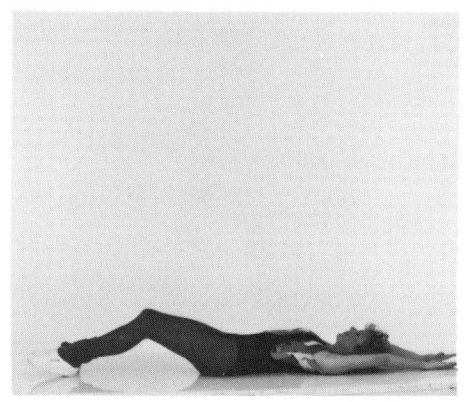 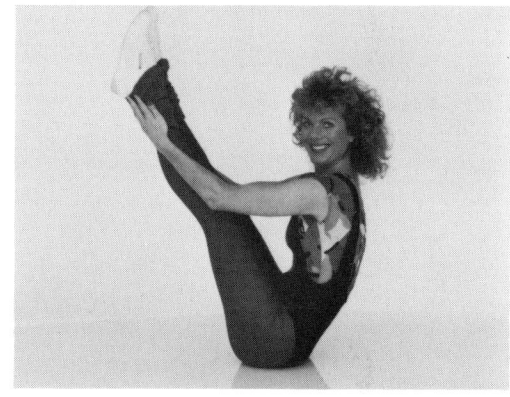

Bring your right leg back to centre, cross your left leg over it and continue the flow of the exercise. Feel the tummy muscles working as you raise and cross the legs. Repeat the sequence.

Lie flat on the floor, arms over your head, legs slightly drawn up. →

In one move, try to sit up, the two halves of the body coming up to meet in the middle. Raise your arms and legs at the same time and finish by balancing on your bottom, holding your ankles. Lie flat and repeat. You can see why this is called the 'Jack Knife'!

Saturday

WARM UP

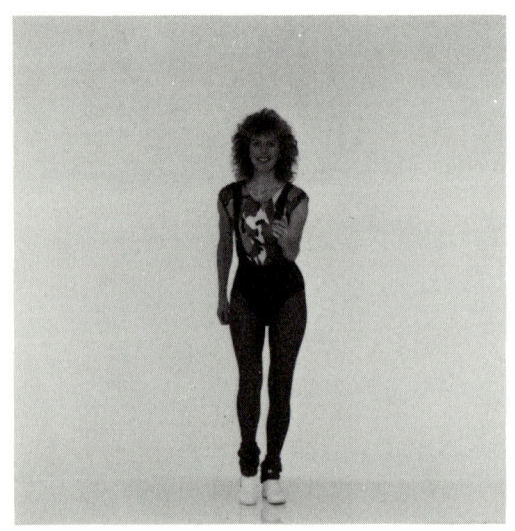 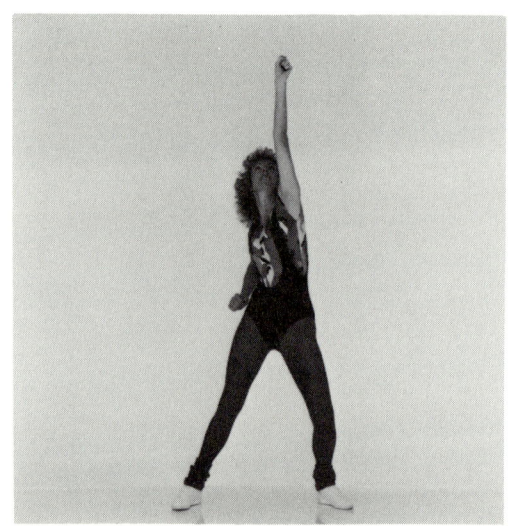 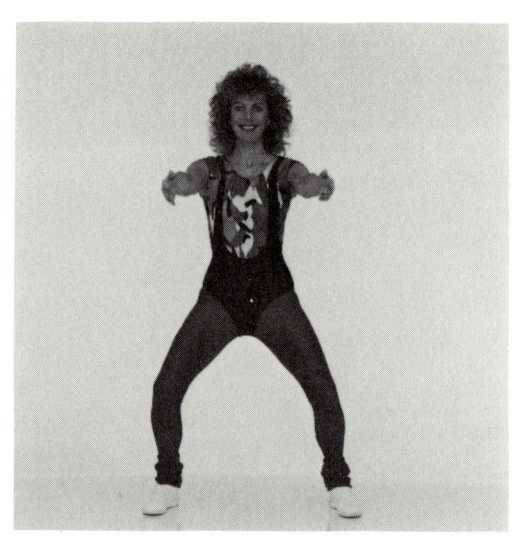

This is a 'miniature' version of marching. Lightly push through each foot, raising each a little off the ground, swinging the arms.

With your legs a comfortable distance apart, raise your right arm, hand in a fist, and bend your right leg. Lower your arm and repeat on the left side. These movements should flow together.

Bend both legs, feet flat on the floor, toes facing front, arms outstretched. Hold that position, straighten up and repeat.

SATURDAY: WARM UP

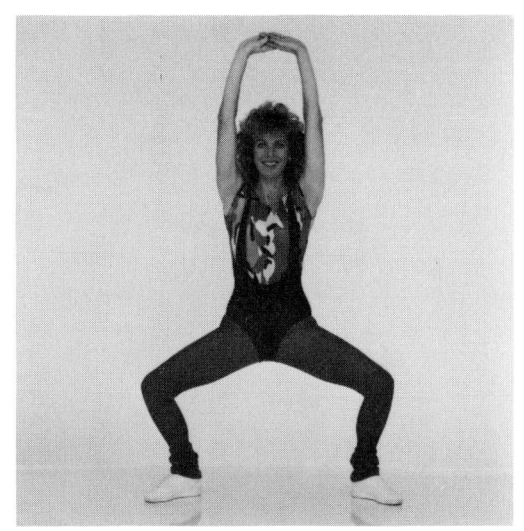 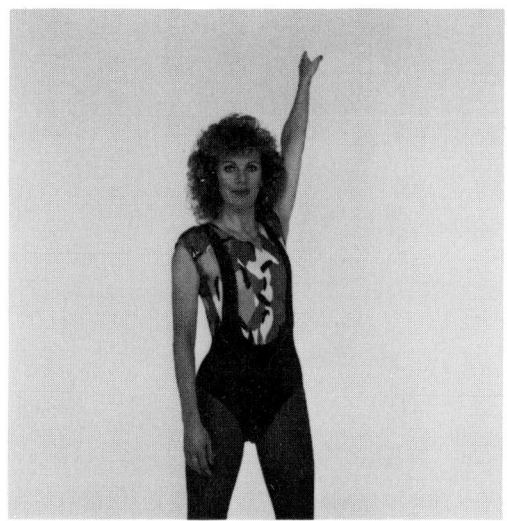 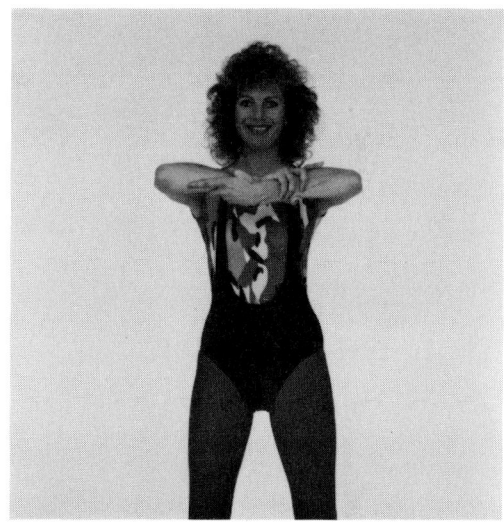

Turn the feet outwards so that the toes point out to their respective diagonals. Clasp your hands together, palms upward, and straighten your arms above your head. Bend your legs, tuck your bottom in and hold that position. Relax — then have another go!

Moving from the shoulder, circle your right arm forward and round in a continuous, flowing movement. Repeat with your left arm.

Bend your arms in front at chest height and hold each wrist with the opposite hand. Gripping the wrists, push those hands away from you. Feel those chest and boob muscles working!

SATURDAY: WARM UP

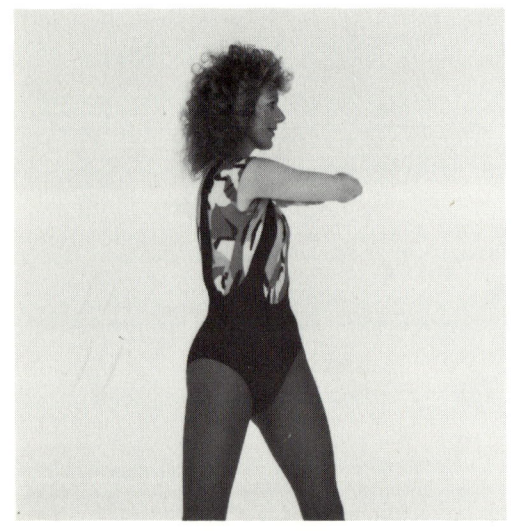 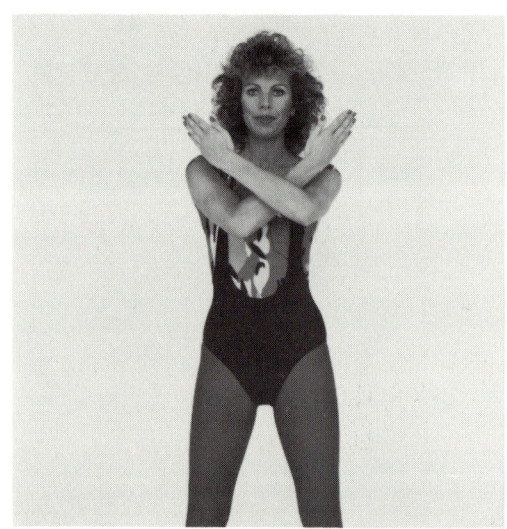 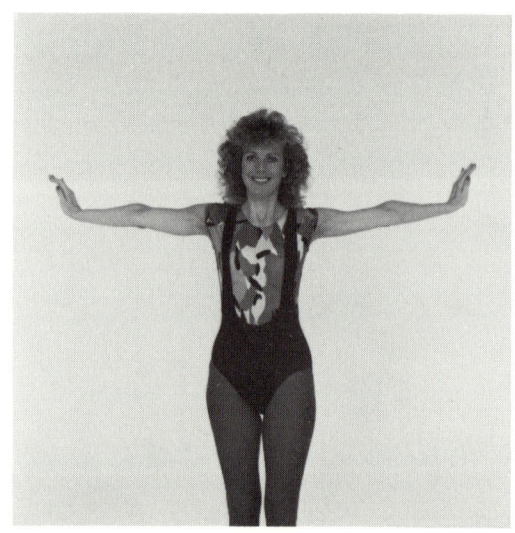

Still holding your wrists in front of you, turn from the waist as far round as you can go, and back to the front. Repeat and then turn to your left.

Start with your arms hanging loosely at your sides and swing them up in front of you so that they cross over at shoulder height. Repeat.

Stretch and straighten your arms out to the sides, fingers pointing to the ceiling. In large, slow circles, guide your arms and shoulders up and around — but keep those arms straight!

SATURDAY: WARM UP

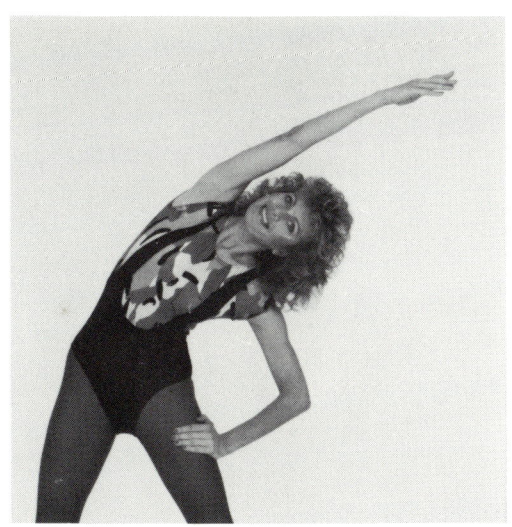 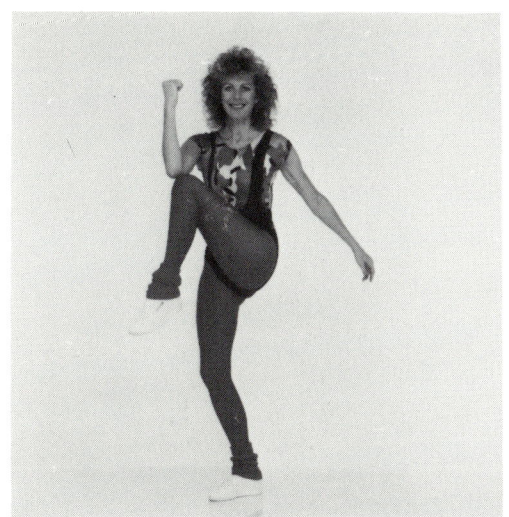 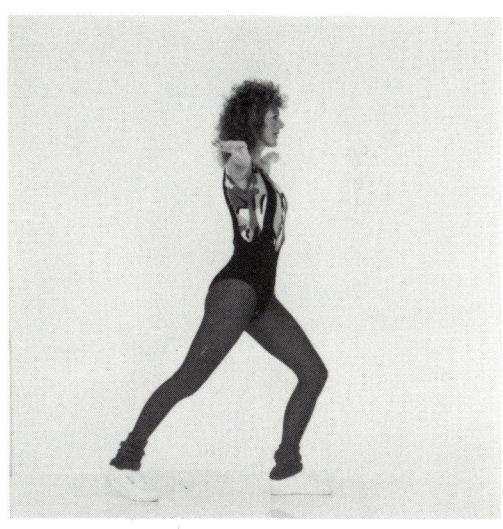

Bend your legs a little as you place your right hand at the top of your thigh. Raise your left arm and curve it over your head, reaching over as far as you can. Enjoy the stretch. Change arms and stretch over to your left.

Raise your right knee across your body and aim to touch it with your left elbow. Don't lean — keep upright. Lower the leg and repeat as many times as you can before changing legs.

Lunge to your right side, bending your right leg, foot flat on the floor, and extending your left leg behind you, arms outstretched at the side for balance. Hold this position, then turn to face your left and repeat.

SATURDAY: HIPS, THIGHS AND BOTTOM STAGE III

HIPS, THIGHS AND BOTTOM STAGE III

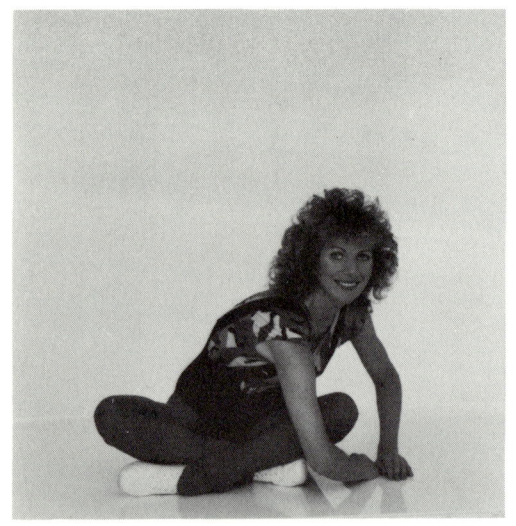
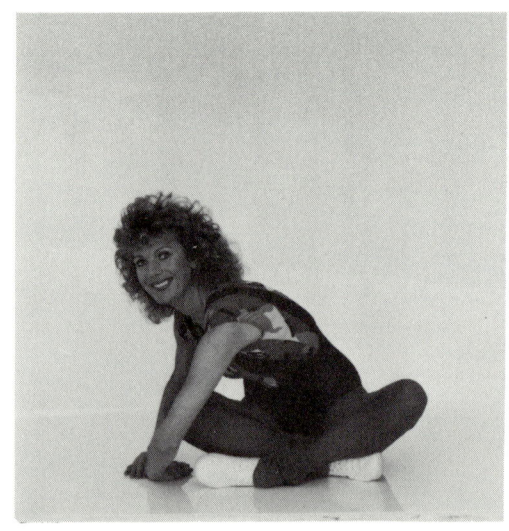
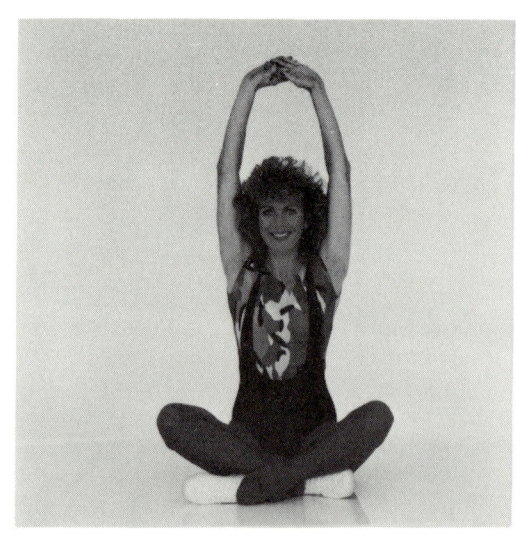

Sit cross-legged on the floor, letting the knees fall outwards. Turning from your waist, place (or attempt to!) both hands flat on the floor to your right. →

Sit up and repeat the exercise to your left.

Still sitting cross-legged, clasp both hands above your head and hold that stretch.

SATURDAY: HIPS, THIGHS AND BOTTOM STAGE III

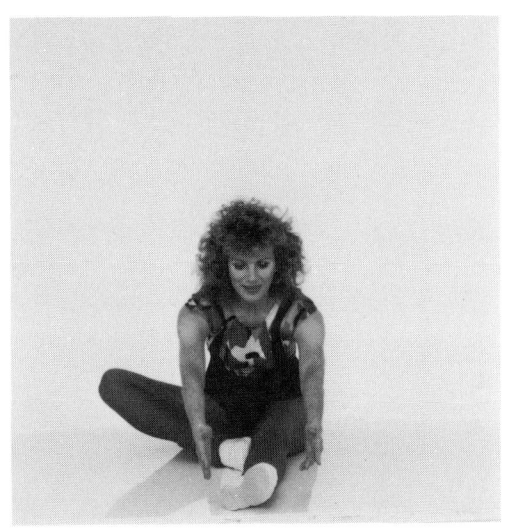 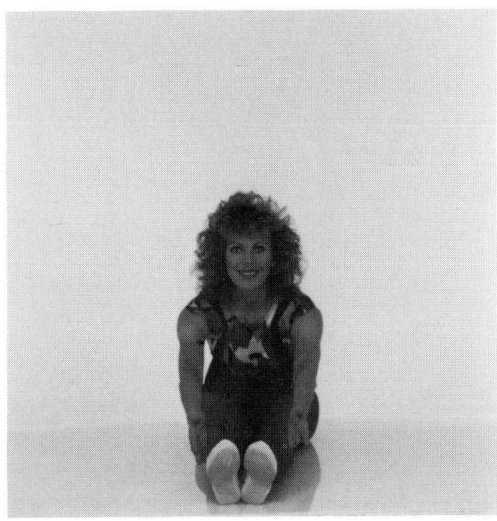 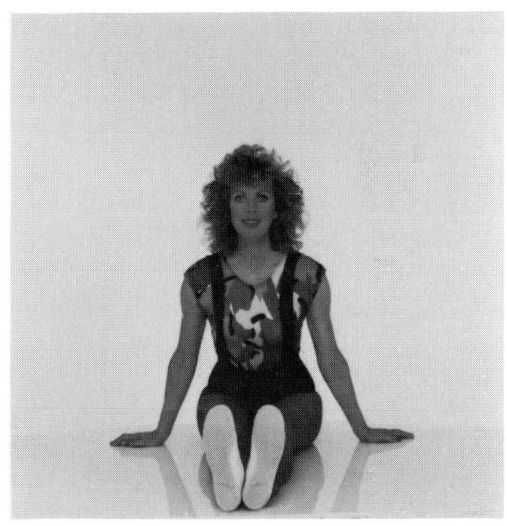

Place your right leg straight in front of you on the floor. Bend your left leg so that your left foot is flat against the inside of your right thigh, knee out. Gently reach forward, easing out of the back of the right leg. Change sides.

With both legs outstretched, gently reach forward, toes pointing down.

This time, point both feet up to the ceiling and place your hands either side on the floor. Keep your back straight as you ease your torso forward and keep upright.

SATURDAY: HIPS, THIGHS AND BOTTOM STAGE III

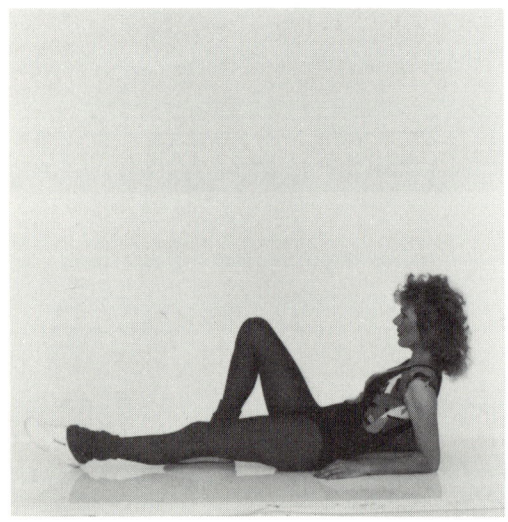

Lie back on your elbows. Bend your right leg, keeping the foot flat on the floor. →

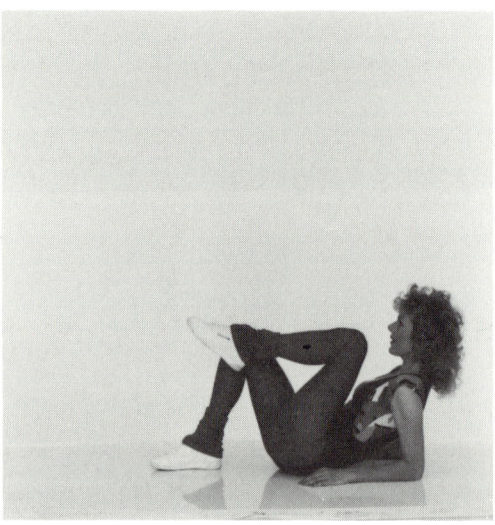

Bend your left knee back towards your chin. →

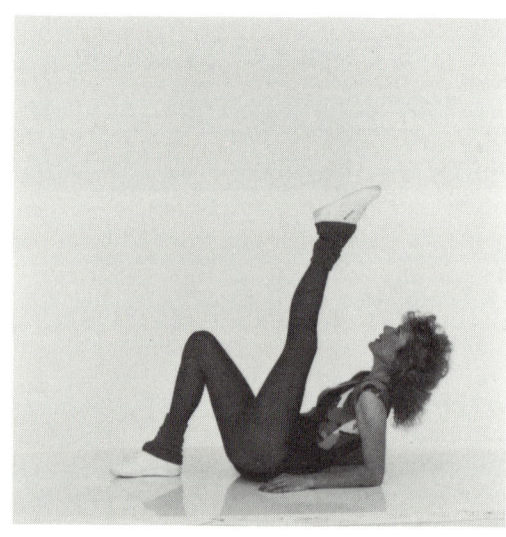

Then lower your left leg straight back down on to the floor, and kick it straight up in the air. Lower. Repeat these movements and change legs.

SATURDAY: HIPS, THIGHS AND BOTTOM STAGE III

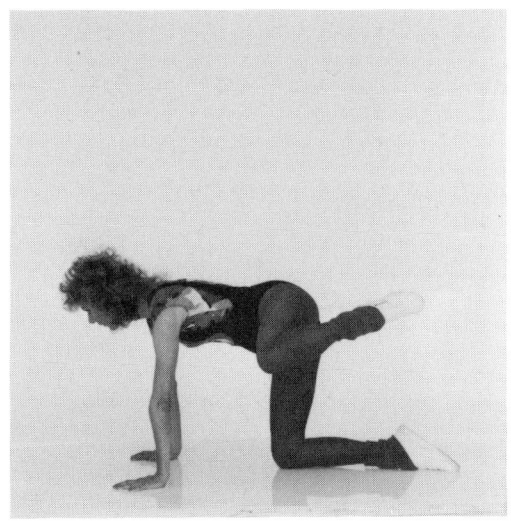 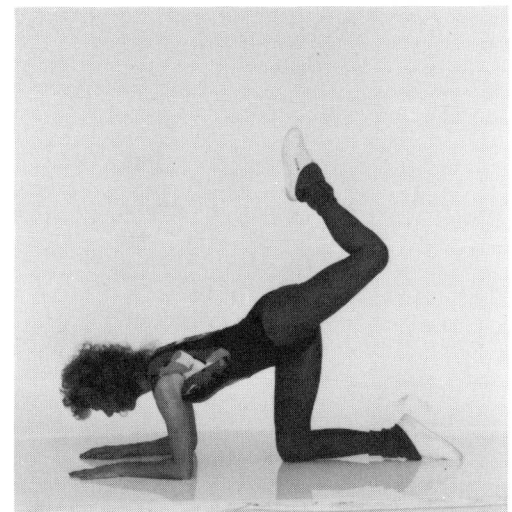 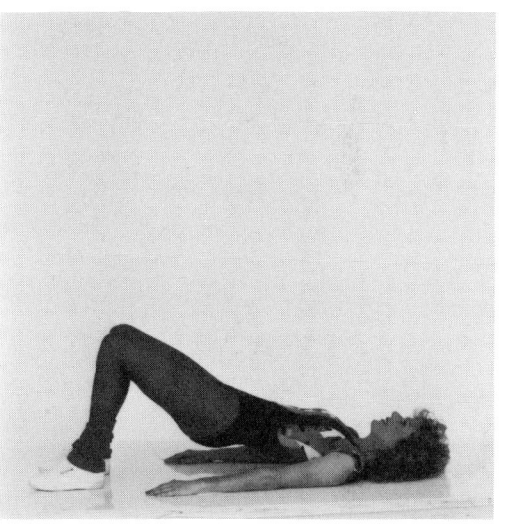

Get down on all fours. Bend your left leg out to your side, raise it as high as you can, keeping it bent, and bring it back in. Change legs and repeat.

Still down on all fours, lower yourself down on to your elbows. Keeping your left leg bent take it as high as you can up behind you. When you bring it back down, keep your knee off the floor. Repeat and change legs. If you feel that this puts too much strain on your back, then leave this exercise out.

Lie flat on your back, knees bent and a small distance apart. Tilt your pelvis but *don't* arch your back as you lift your bottom off the floor. Hold that position and tense the muscles in your buttocks. Relax back into the floor. Repeat.

SATURDAY: LEG EXERCISES STAGE I

LEG EXERCISES STAGE I

Exercise undoubtedly gets easier: like any activity, the more familiar you become with the subject, the quicker you will understand and progress — as long as you do it regularly! Power in the leg muscles is not only built up with a variety of exercises but also with the repetition of the same exercises. These leg exercises are a repeat of yesterday's — but today you should find that you can achieve more.

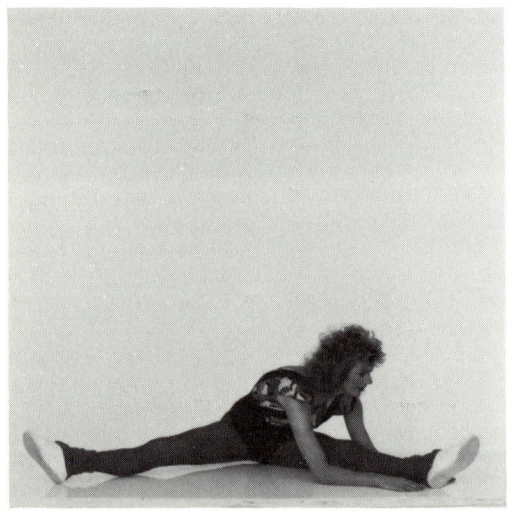 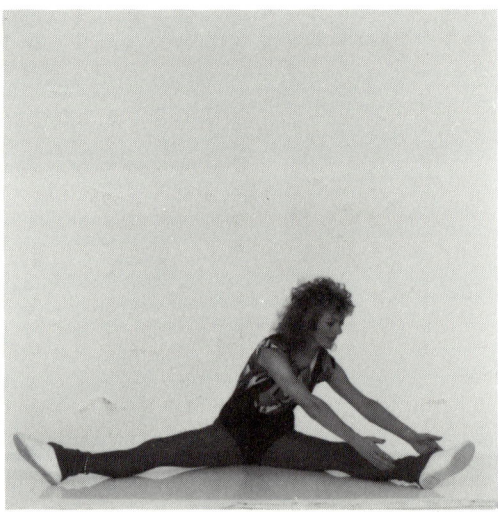 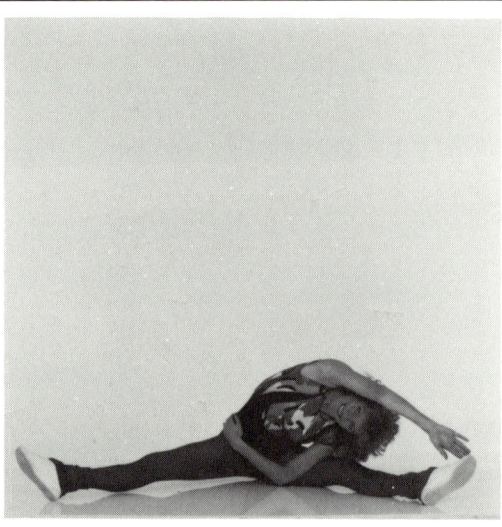

Sit on the floor, legs apart and, turning from the waist, lean your torso directly in line with your right leg. Try not to hunch your back. With a tiny movement, reach forward towards your toes. Change sides and try to your left.

Now try reaching for your toes with both hands, keeping your back straight, tummy in, and hold the stretch. Change sides.

Sit up and raise your left arm over your head, bending your right arm over your body so that it almost touches your left hip. Turn from the waist and reach over with your left arm, aiming to touch your right foot with your left fingers.

SATURDAY: LEG EXERCISES STAGE I

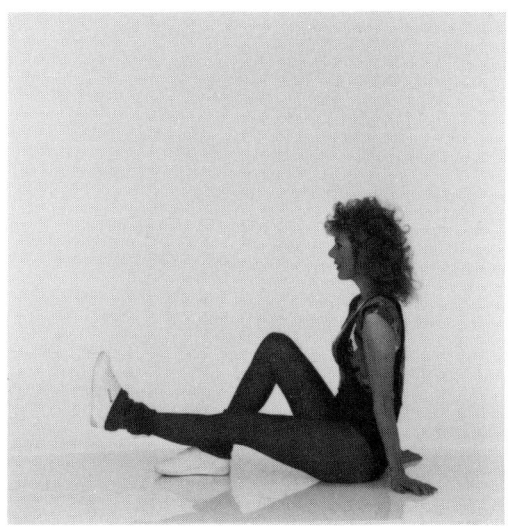
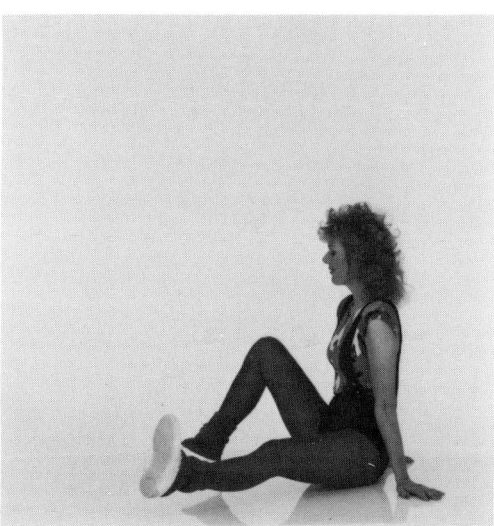
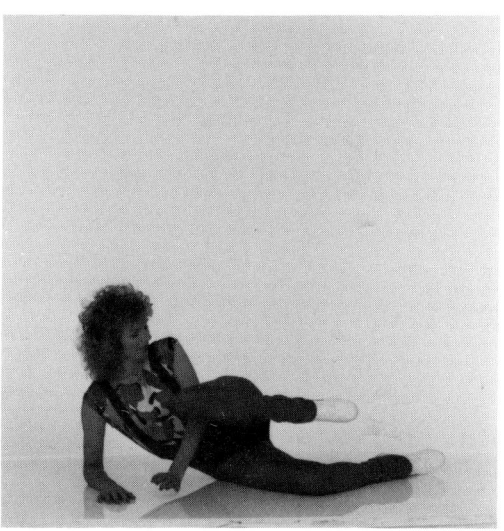

Sit up and place both hands behind you to support your weight. Bend your right leg and keep the foot flat on the floor. Keep your left leg straight out in front, toes pointing to the ceiling, and raise and lower it — keeping it off the floor. Change legs.

From the same starting position as the previous exercise, raise your left leg, open it out to your side and 'swing' it shut. Open and close your right leg, keeping it off the floor. Change legs.

Lie on your left side, bending your left arm and leg underneath you. Raise and bend your right leg up towards your chest. →

SATURDAY: LEG EXERCISES STAGE I

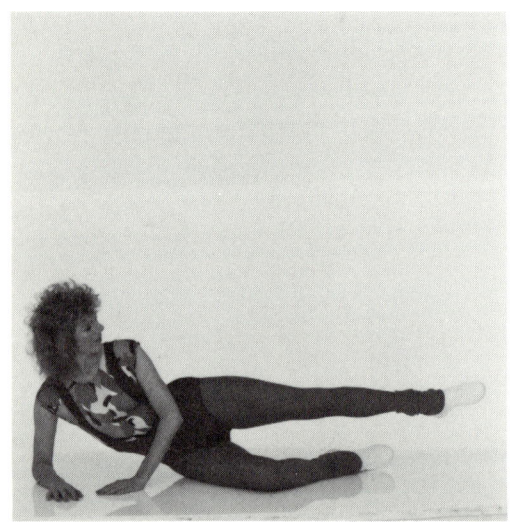
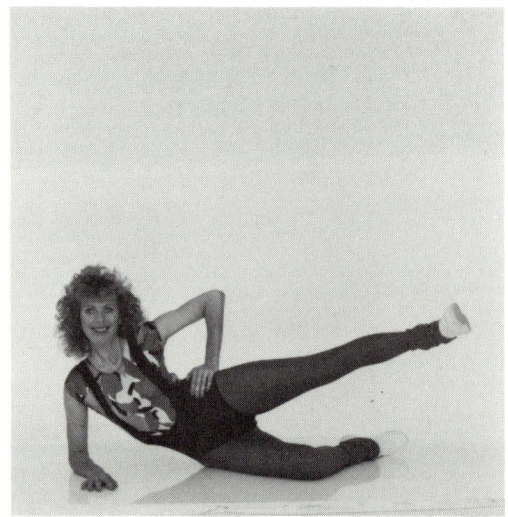
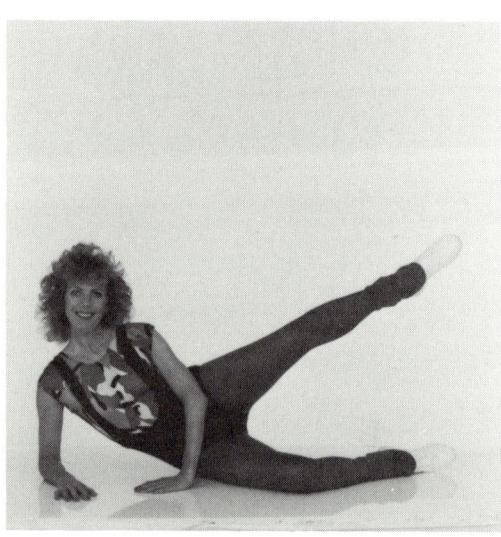

Extend your right leg away from you, off the ground. →

Raise and lower your right leg, keeping the foot flat, toes pointing to the front. Again, keep the foot off the floor as you lower it. →

Bend your right leg and raise and lower it slowly, this time with the toes pointing straight. Now change sides and repeat these four movements, working your left leg.

SATURDAY: LEG EXERCISES STAGE I

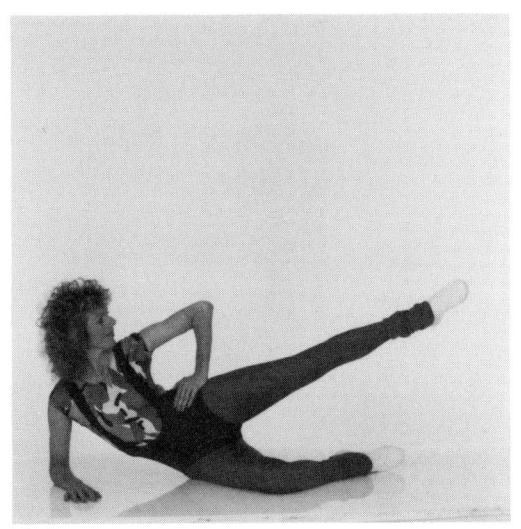

Lie back on your left side, raise your right leg and circle the leg slowly forward and round. 'Draw' large circles in the air. →

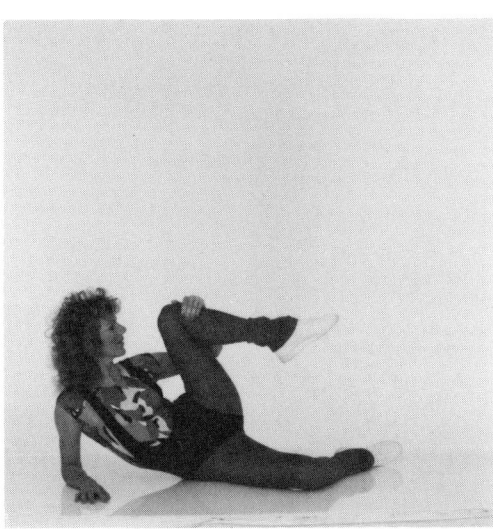

Bend your right knee in so that it points towards your head, and hold it lightly below the kneecap. →

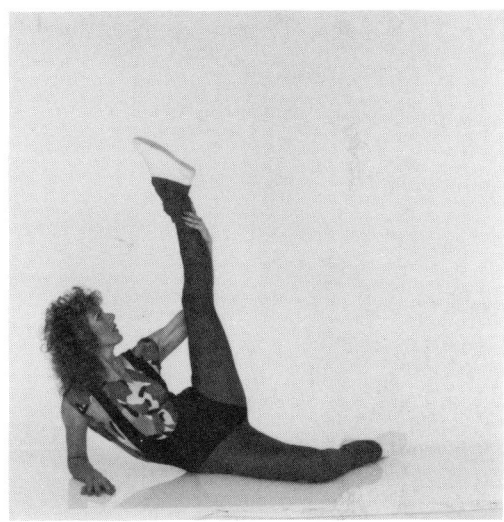

Straighten the leg down, then kick straight up in the air, turning out from the very top of the leg. Catch it below the calf. Repeat these three movements and change sides.

SATURDAY: POP DANCE

POP DANCE

Today's the day you can shine out at your nightclub or party. The dance routine you learned yesterday should be enjoyed today — but to a different rhythm. Choose one of your favourite records and practise the dance sequence. As you become more familiar with the routine you can vary the number of times you do each movement.

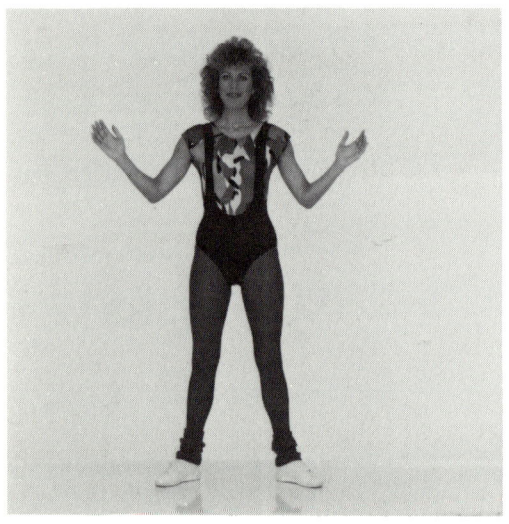

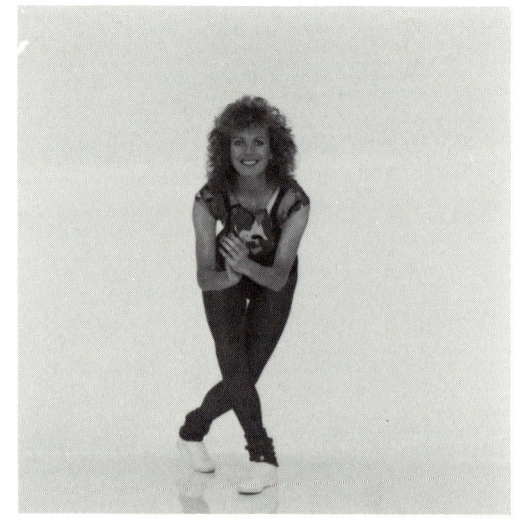

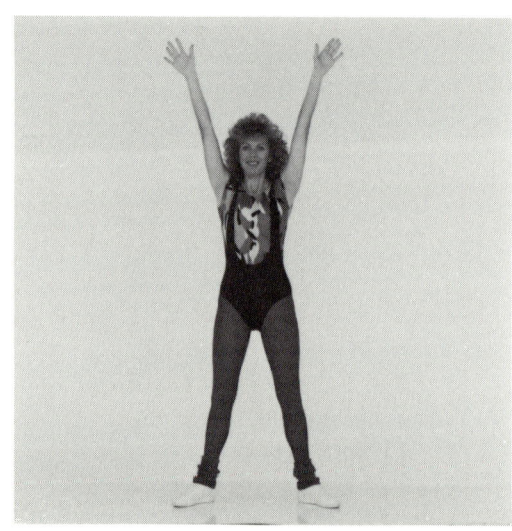

Stand with your feet and legs a comfortable distance apart and your arms open. →

Bend your left leg as you cross your right foot behind it, heel raised. At the same time, clap your hands and crouch forward, head up. →

Stand tall, stretching both arms above your head and step on your right foot. →

SATURDAY: POP DANCE

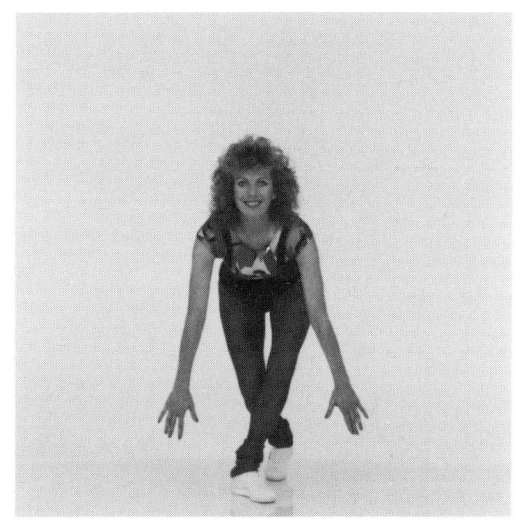 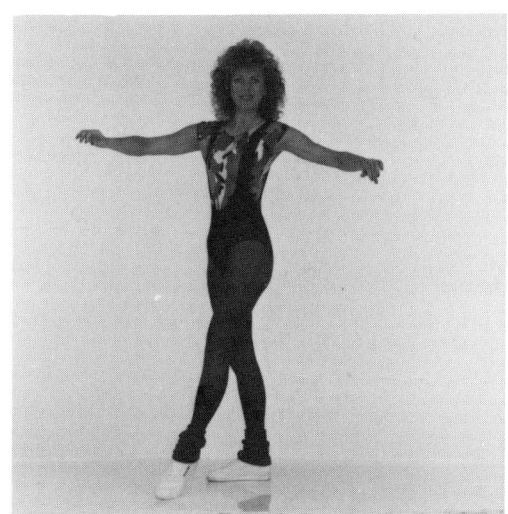 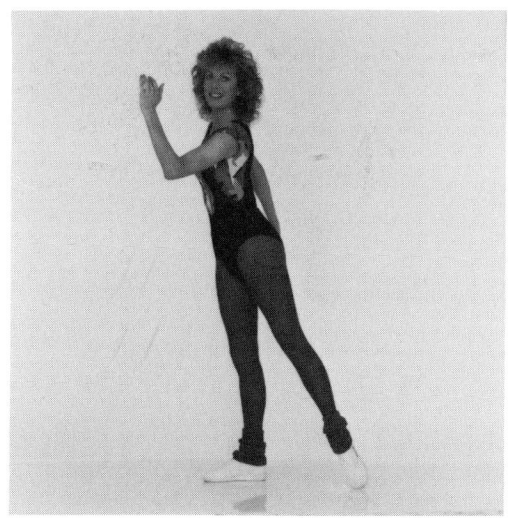

Cross your left foot behind your right, bend both legs and shoot your arms down either side of your body. Keep repeating this sequence.

Turn your body to your left diagonal as you move your right foot in front across your body, toes touching the floor, swing your left arm in front. →

Point your right foot behind, swinging your right arm up in front. Do these two steps four times and repeat using your left leg.

SATURDAY: POP DANCE

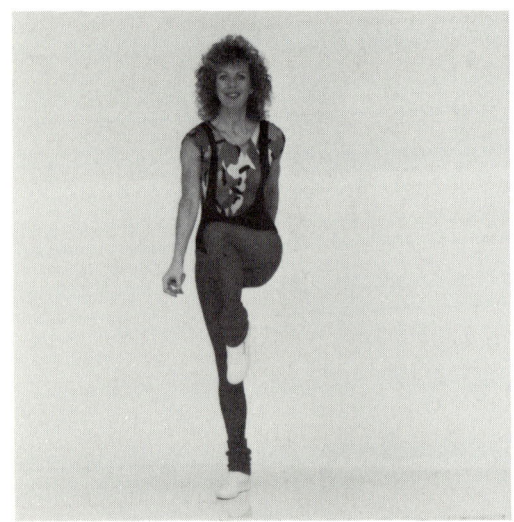

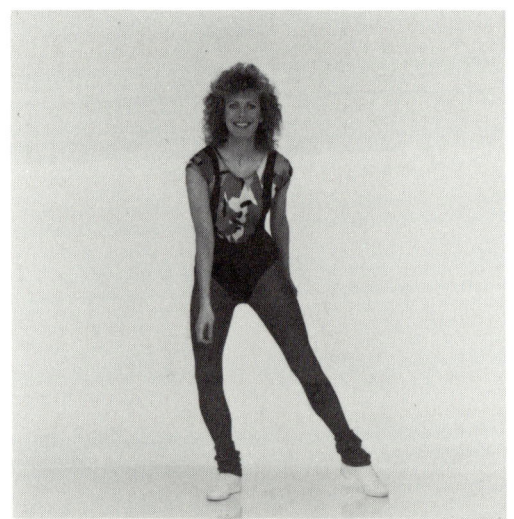

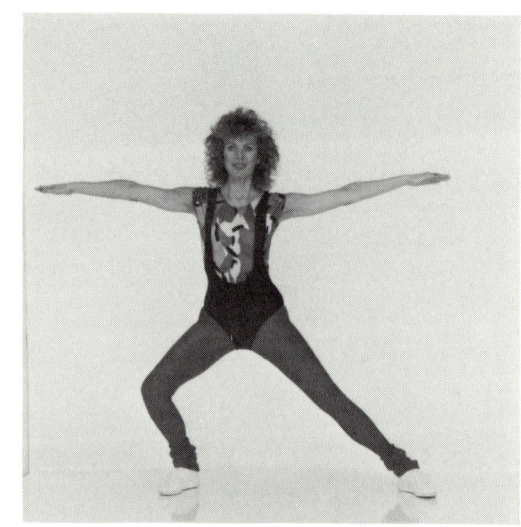

On the next beat quickly face your left diagonal again and jump your right knee up across your body. →

And land lightly, touching the floor with your right foot to the side. Repeat these two movements together four times and then continue, facing your right diagonal, working your left leg.

Slow the pace down by lunging from side to side. Step your left leg to the side and bend it, extending both arms out to your sides. Hold for one beat, then transfer your weight by bending your right leg. Repeat four times each side, holding for one beat between the changes. Now try it in double-time: do eight fast changes, clapping as you change the lunge.

SATURDAY: POP DANCE

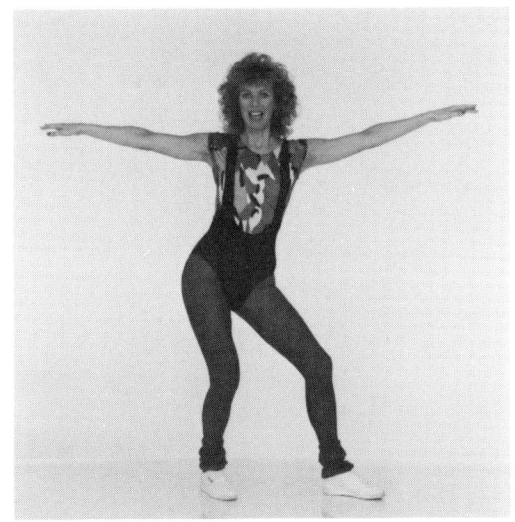 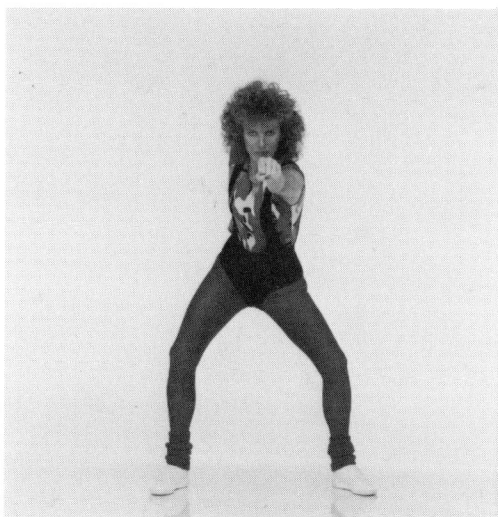 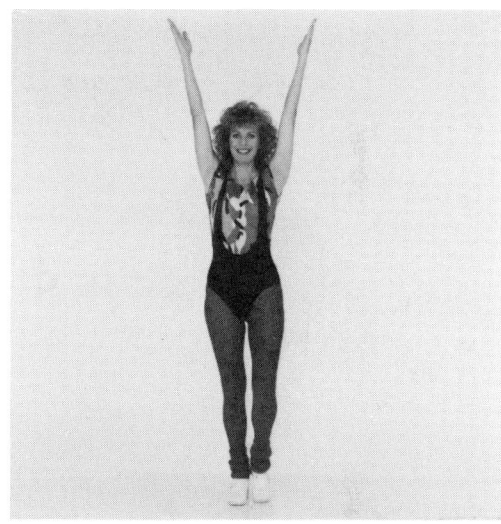

Swing those hips in preparation for tonight's party! Bend both legs and try to do whole circles, guiding your hips round to your left, front, right and behind. Then try swinging them from side to side.

With your feet apart and your legs bent, pretend to shadow-box with a partner. Punch straight in front, through the air, and then do double punches. You can also do this exercise punching straight above your head and alternating each arm — but only single punches.

To finish off, get on the move again. Lightly marking time with a tiny jogging movement, raise both arms above your head, open them wide and clap your hands sixteen times.

Sunday

WARM UP

This is the day you probably have more time to think about *you*, more time to devote to yourself, so why not enjoy a constructive Sunday and set your goals really high with these exercises. If you have some extra time attempt each exercise twelve times.

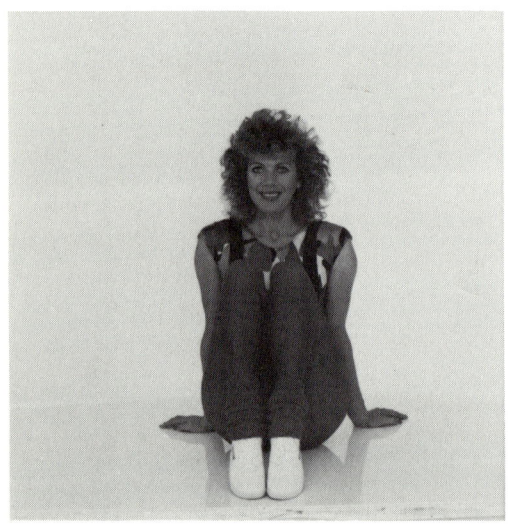

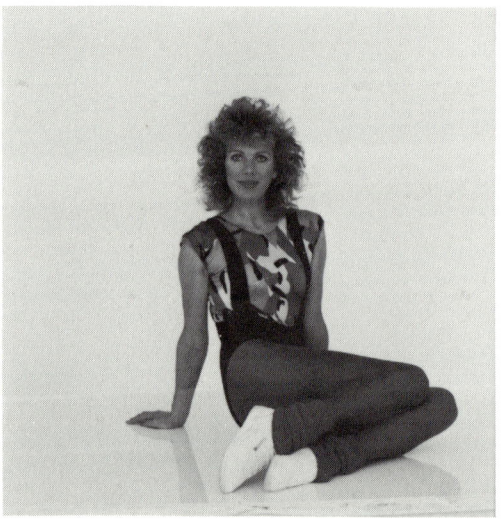

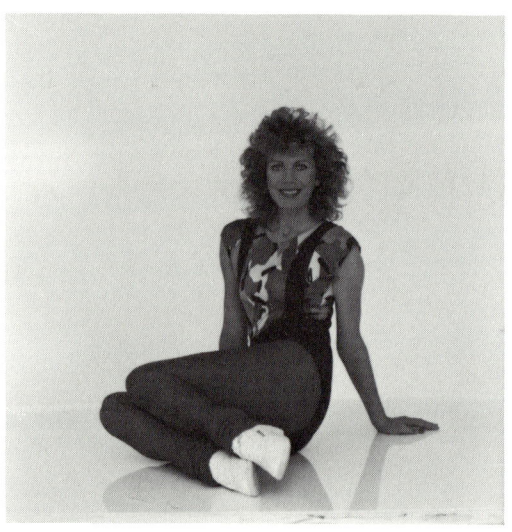

Sit on the floor, hands on the floor either side. Draw your knees up, toes pointing on the floor. Sit up. →

Keeping your legs together, let both knees roll across your body so that your right knee comes down to touch the floor. Try to keep your torso facing front so that you are working from the waist. Bring both legs back to the centre. →

And repeat to your left.

SUNDAY: WARM UP

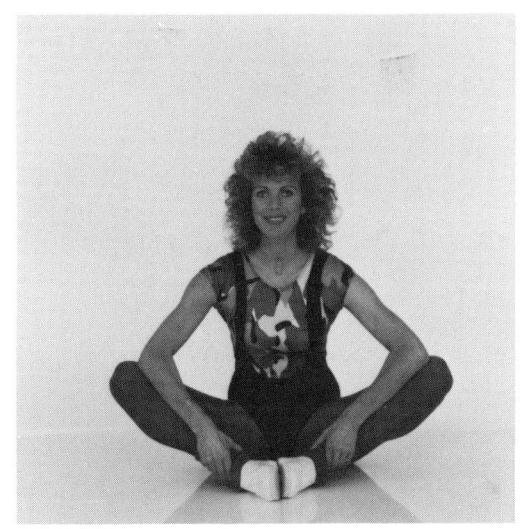 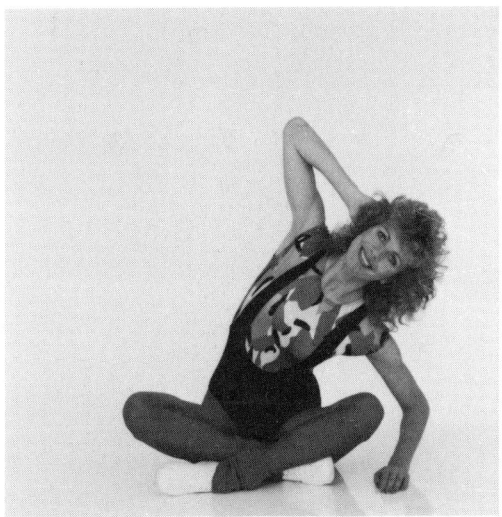 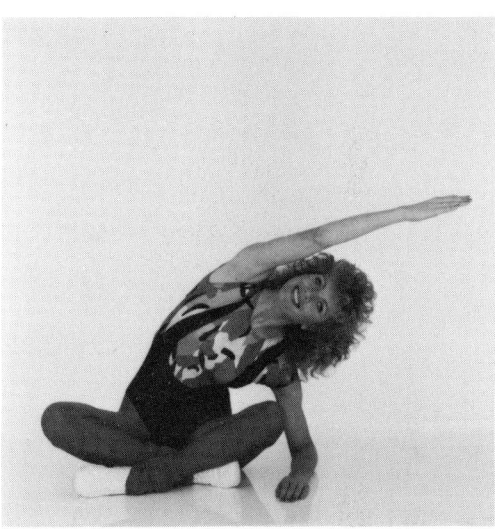

Sit with your knees flopping out, soles of the feet touching. Grasp both ankles and, with the help of your hands, practise correct posture by 'sitting tall' and then collapsing into the centre.

Sitting cross-legged, place your right hand on the floor, bend your left arm and rest the fingers lightly on the side of your head and lean to your right side. Keep your left elbow pointing upwards and gently reach over eight times. Change arms and lean to your left.

This time curve your whole arm over your head and lower on to your right forearm. Change arms and stretch over with your right arm.

SUNDAY: WARM UP

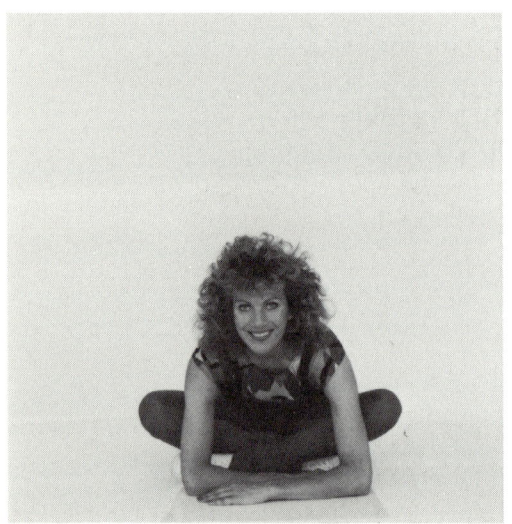
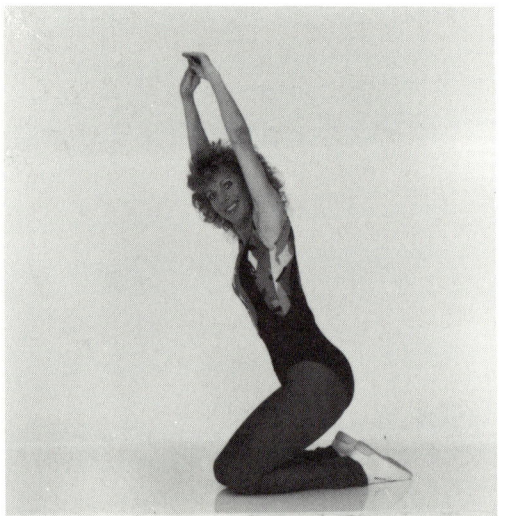
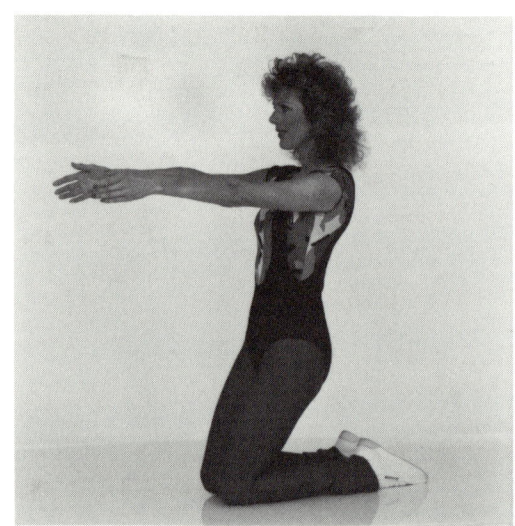

You might not be able to do this fully, but see how far you can lean forward. Sitting cross-legged, place your hands on the floor in front of you. Gently flatten your back as you lower yourself on to your forearms — *don't* over-stretch.

Kneel down and clasp your hands above your head. Raise your bottom so that you are not sitting on your feet. Circle the hips and bottom by sinking round to the right — just above the feet — and coming up again round to the left. Repeat, circling the other way.

Kneeling upright, arms outstretched in front, slowly lean back — don't do a back bend — *lean* the torso back, keeping the back straight. Feel the stretch on the thighs, and slowly come forward again.

SUNDAY: WARM UP

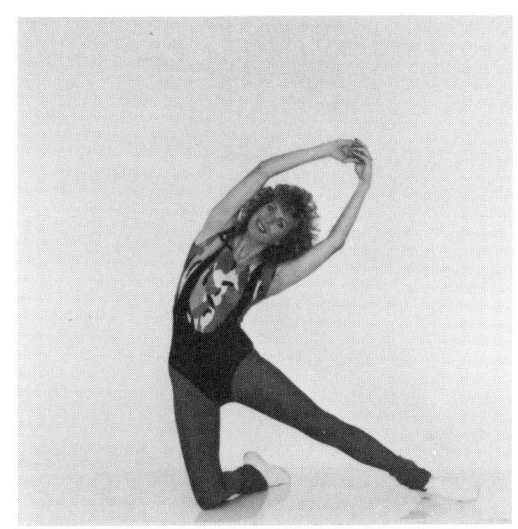 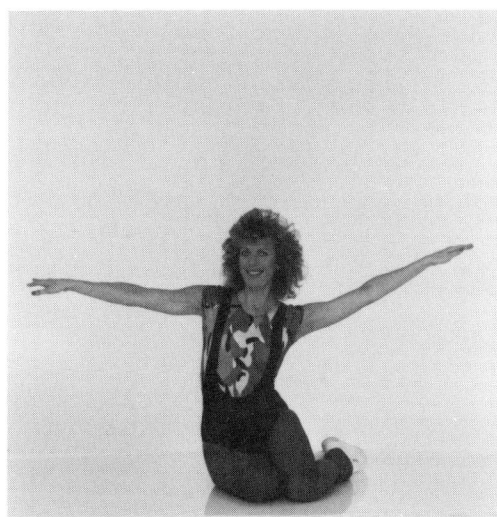 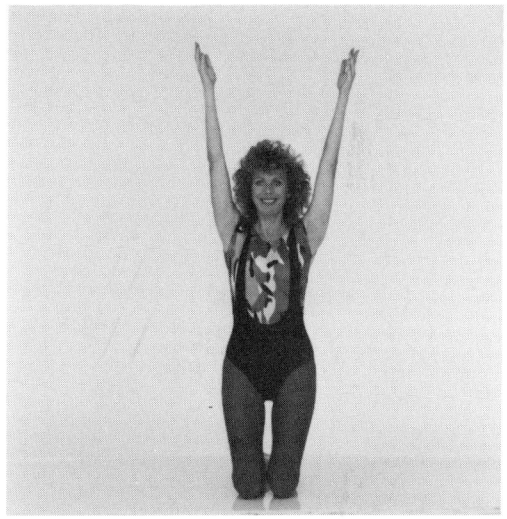

Kneel on your left leg and extend your right leg to the side. Holding your hands above your head, lean to the right. With a tiny movement reach over eight times. Change legs and lean to your left.

Sit with both legs bent and tucked under your right side, arms stretched out either side. Lean towards your right. →

Now try swooping your arms forward and up as you push up through your thighs on to your knees. This action is one single movement and you might not achieve it to begin with, your thighs need to be strong and your balance and coordination good. Come down from the kneeling position with both legs bent and tucked under your left side. Lean to your left and repeat.

SUNDAY: CHAIR EXERCISES

CHAIR EXERCISES

For those of you who particularly enjoy the chair exercises, and as Sunday is traditionally a day of rest, you can finish reading the Sunday newspapers whilst gently exercising! Perhaps today you can attempt a little more as you are probably feeling nice and relaxed.

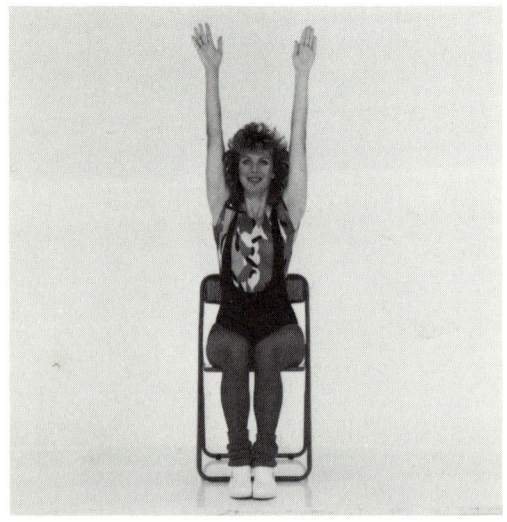

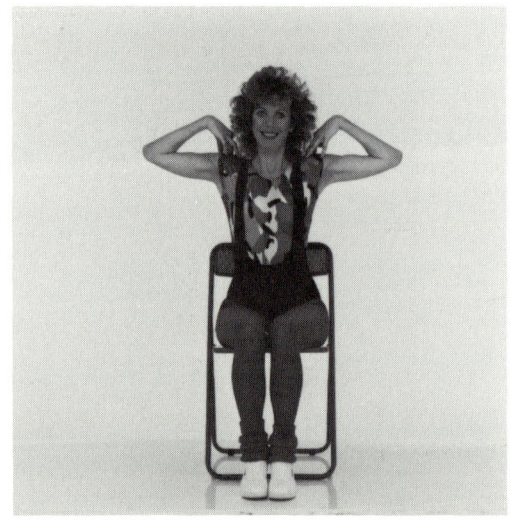

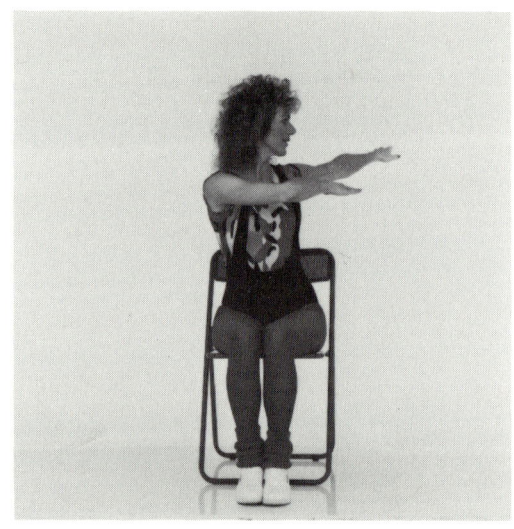

Have a good stretch and reach up to fill that space.

Place your hands on your shoulders and, guided by your elbows, circle your shoulders up and round. Reverse the circle.

Bend your left arm in front of you at chest height. Extend your right arm to the side and, turning from the waist, ease your torso round to the right. Bring your arms back to the front and reverse the exercise, bending your right arm, extending your left and turning to your left.

SUNDAY: CHAIR EXERCISES

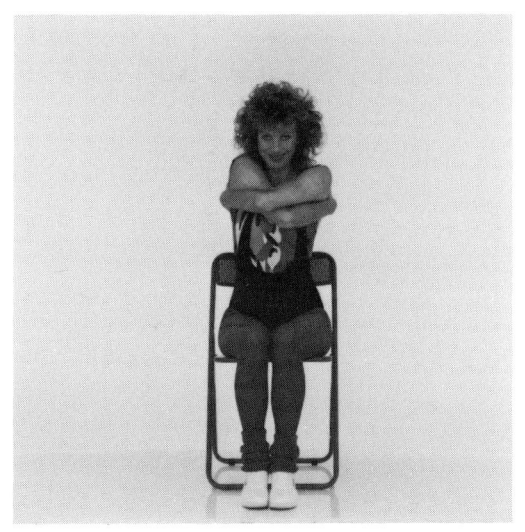

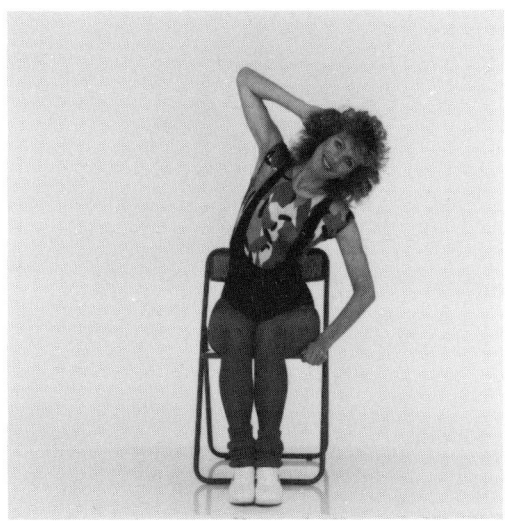

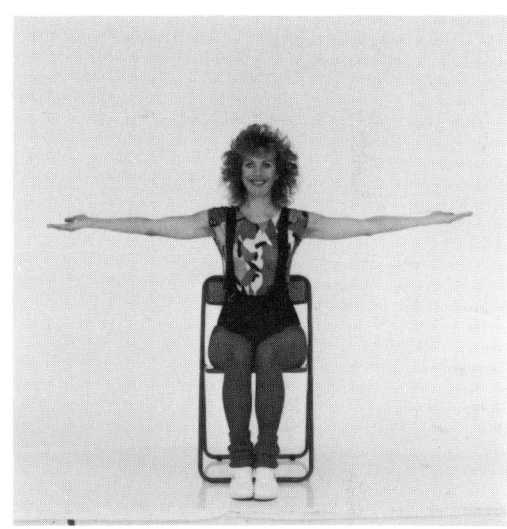

Hug yourself! Wrap your arms around your body, shoulders up. Unfold and try again: see how far you can reach round with your fingertips.

Place your right hand on the side of the chair for balance. Place your left hand at the side of your head, elbow up to the ceiling. Lean directly over to your right. Centralize, change hands and lean to your left.

Stretch both arms out to your sides and, with a twisting movement, turn both arms up and over. Keep your arms straight.

SUNDAY: CHAIR EXERCISES

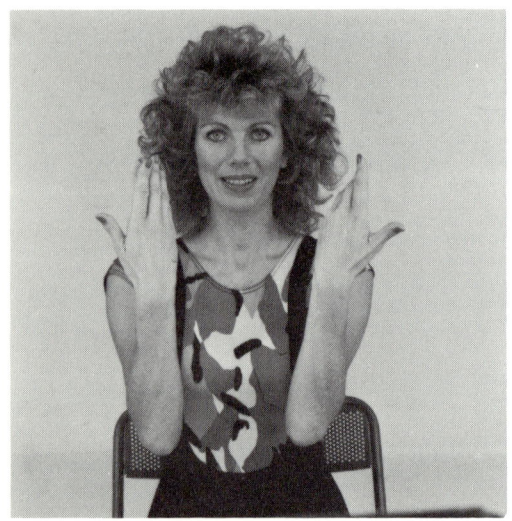
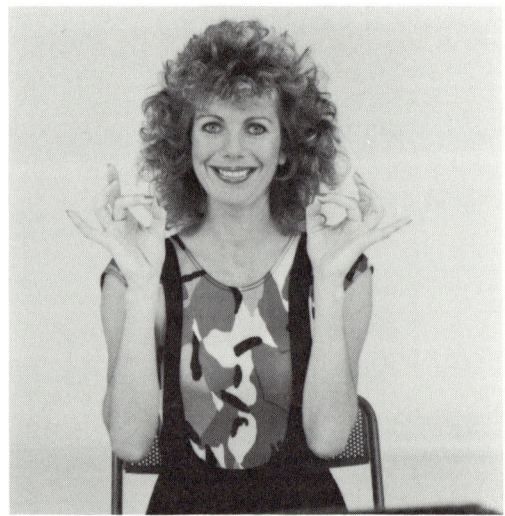
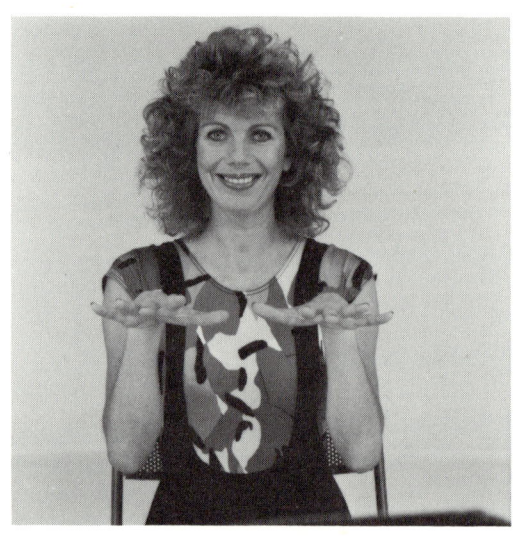

Bend your arms in front of you, elbows down, and circle both hands round away from each other and then back.

Touch your thumb with each finger — the tip of the finger should touch the tip of your thumb. Do this continuously, working from the little finger to the index finger and out again.

With both hands in front of you, palms down, make a fist, then splay the fingers out, spreading and stretching them, and make a fist again.

SUNDAY: CHAIR EXERCISES

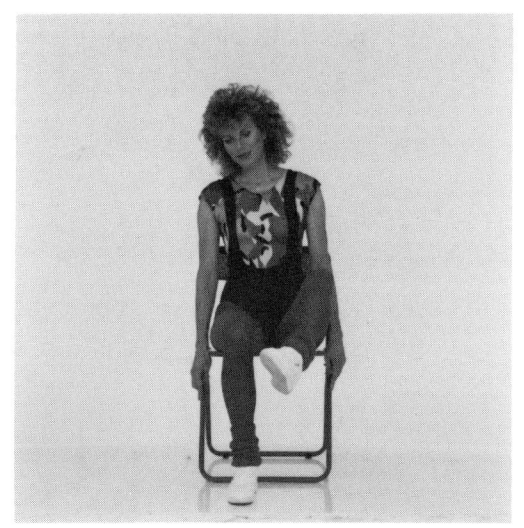 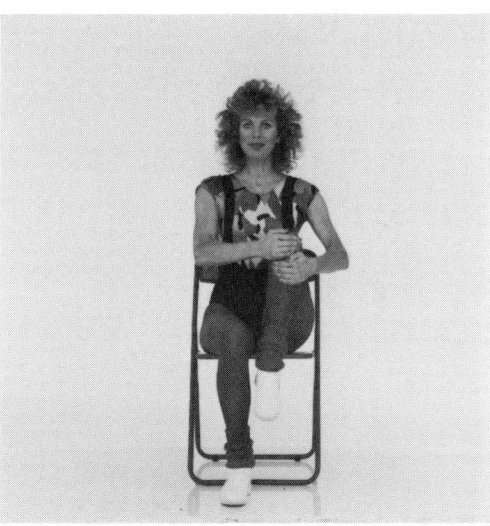 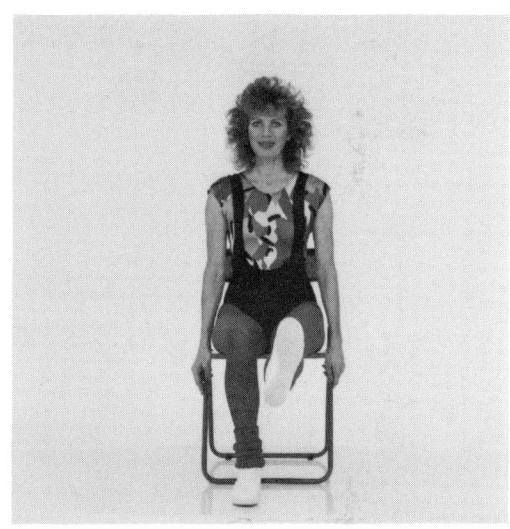

Raise your right foot and draw large, continuous circles in the air, clockwise and anticlockwise. Change feet.

Hug your right knee, holding it just below the knee, and ease it up. →

Extend the leg straight in front, foot up, toes pointing to the ceiling, and lower. Repeat and change feet.

SUNDAY: LEG EXERCISES STAGE II

LEG EXERCISES STAGE II

This is a combination of standing exercises followed by the hardest floor exercises. After a few weeks you will find these exercises much easier — no longer will phrases like 'weak at the knees' and 'my legs turned to jelly' apply to you!

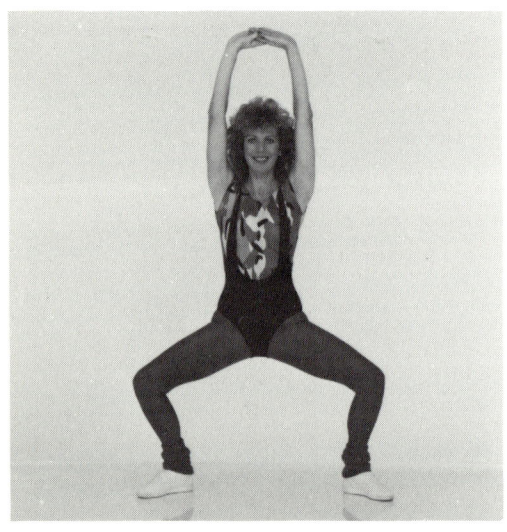 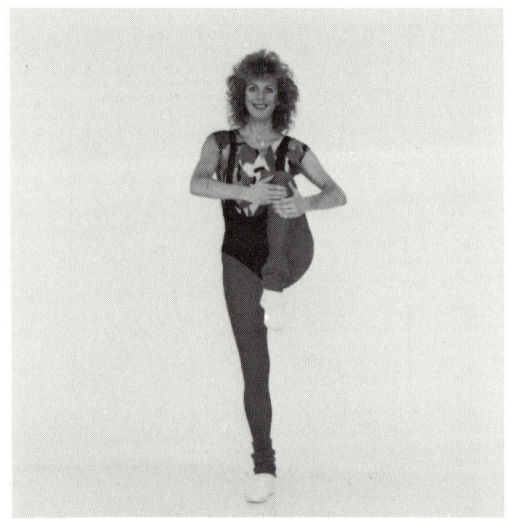 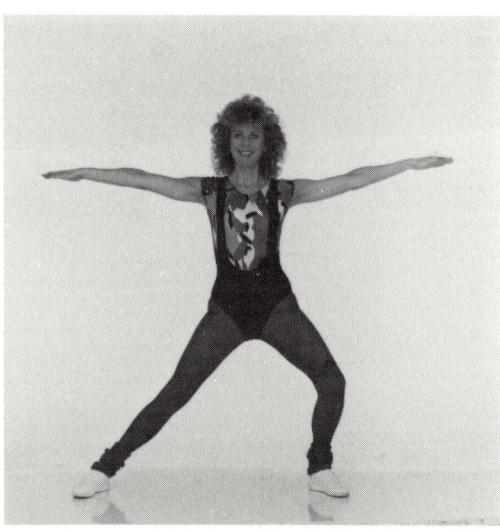

Stand with your legs and feet a comfortable distance apart, feet flat on the floor. Bend your legs, and as you do so raise your arms above your head, clasping your fingers together. Hold this position. Lower your arms and straighten your legs. Repeat this four times.

Standing straight, bring your right knee up towards your chest and hug it lightly. Repeat with your left knee and continue alternating each leg in rhythm. Attempt 10–20.

Bend your right leg and extend your left leg out to the side — but don't turn your foot out, keep the toes facing forward. For balance, raise your arms out to your sides. →

SUNDAY: LEG EXERCISES STAGE II

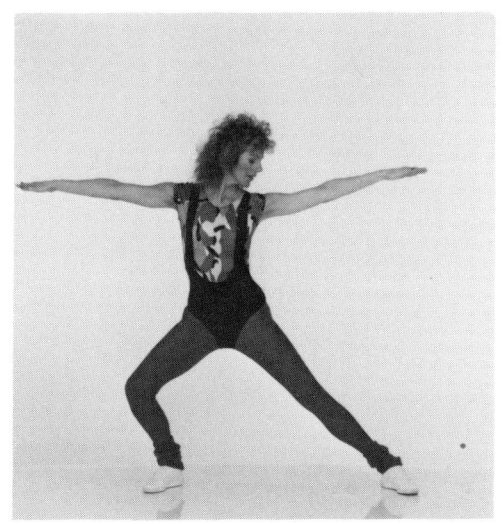 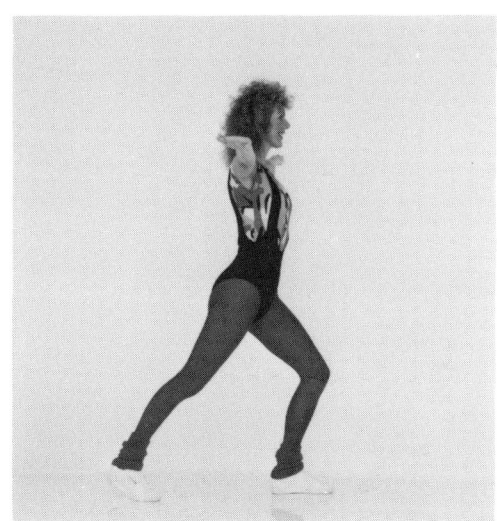 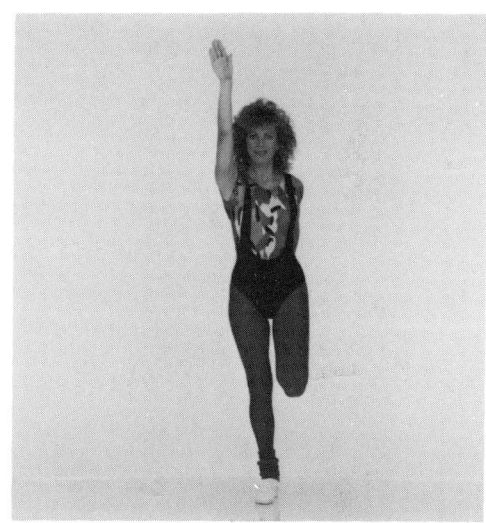

Reverse the exercise by swinging through to bend your left leg, thereby straightening the right. Transfer the weight, working right through each leg, sixteen times.

Facing your right, lunge forward and step on a bent right leg, arms out to your sides. Straighten up, face front and repeat to your left, lunging on to a bent left leg. Repeat this movement eight times on each side.

Balancing on your left leg, bend your right leg behind you so that you can hold your right foot with your right hand, feel the stretch on your right thigh. Hold for 30 seconds and change legs.

SUNDAY: LEG EXERCISES STAGE II

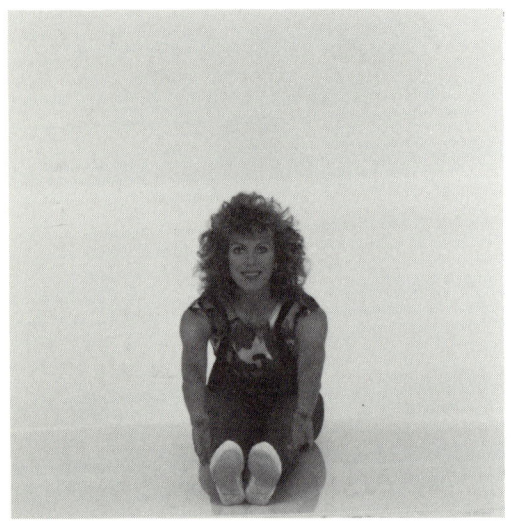

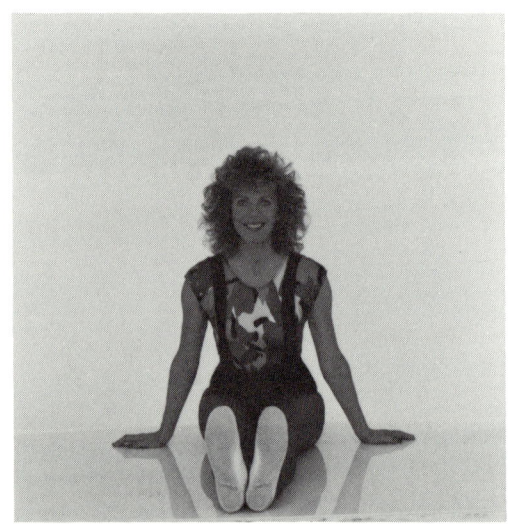

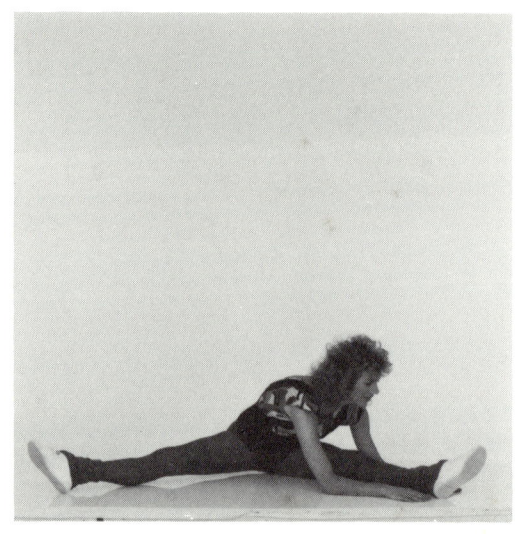

Sit on the floor, feet and legs together, toes pointed. Keeping your back flat, reach forward with minimal movements towards your feet.

Place your hands flat on the floor at your sides and point your toes up towards the ceiling. Sitting up straight, gently lean forward with tiny movements. Repeat.

Sit with your legs wide apart — but keep that distance comfortable. Turn from your waist so that your torso is in line with your right leg and lean down as low as you can over your leg for as long as you can. Rise up, turn from your waist, line up with your left leg and over you go!

SUNDAY: LEG EXERCISES STAGE II

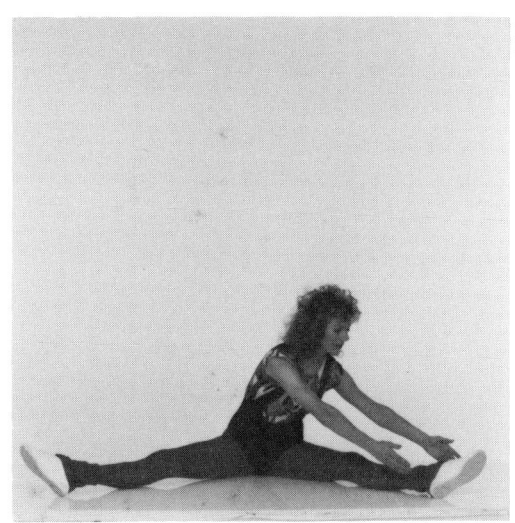 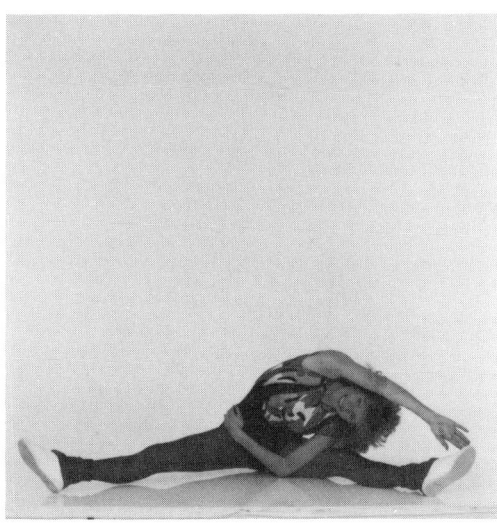 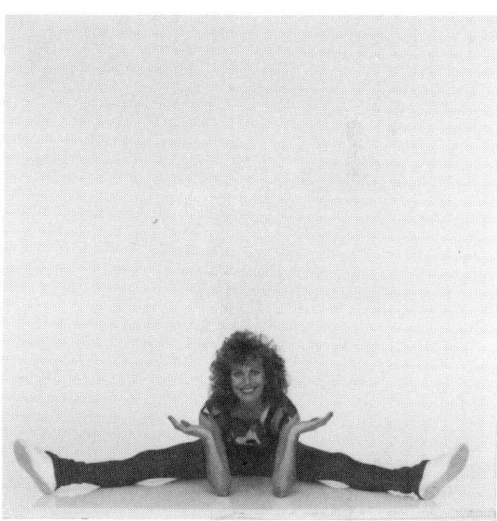

Sit with your legs wide apart, but this time keep your back straight as you reach forward with both arms, first towards your right toes, then your left.

Again, legs wide apart, raise your left arm over your head and turn sideways over your right leg, reaching down as low as you can. Centralize and repeat to your right.

Complete Sunday's leg exercises by gently stretching the insides of the thighs. Flatten your back and put your elbows on the floor in front of you . . . one day you will!

So How Are You Doing?

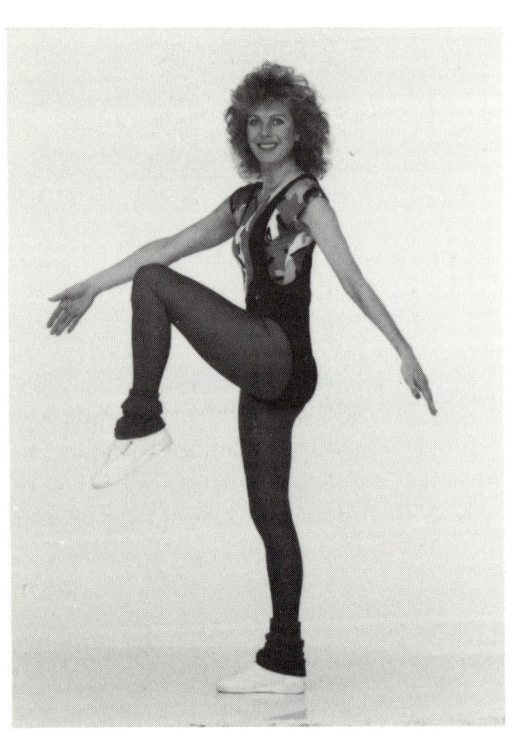

It is so satisfying to feel the benefits of regular exercise — and see the difference! Chart your progress by repeating these tests once a week and, if you fill in your progress chart on a monthly basis, you will notice how much more you are achieving and how much better you feel!

SO HOW ARE YOU DOING?

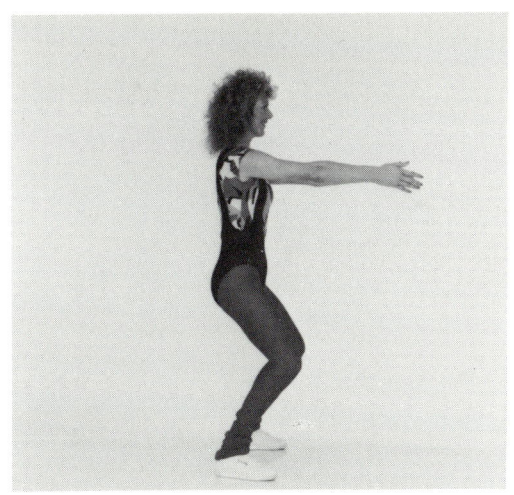 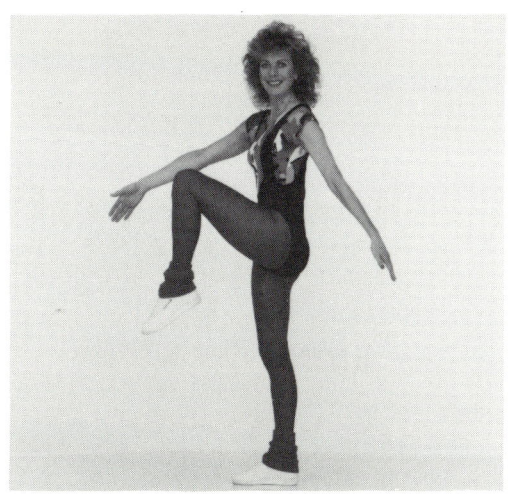 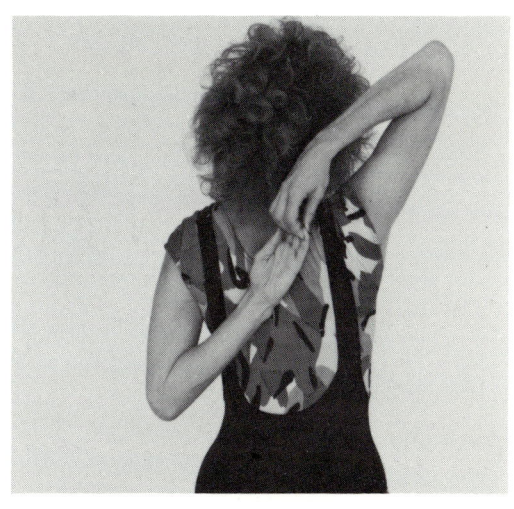

THIGH HOLD
Stand with your feet and legs a comfortable distance apart, toes facing front, arms outstretched in front, directly in line with your legs. Bend your legs, keeping your feet flat on the floor. How long can you hold this position? Straighten up and relax as soon as your thighs feel any strain, and shake out the legs. Now repeat this test, this time with your toes pointed out a little. ULTIMATE ACHIEVEMENT: ONE MINUTE

HIGH MARCHING
Raising each leg as high as possible, march on the spot. Swing your arms as you do when walking — the opposite arm to the raised leg. Control your foot as it comes down, don't crash it down on the floor, lightly place and work through the foot to raise each leg. ULTIMATE ACHIEVEMENT: 80–100 PACES

SHOULDER SUPPLENESS
Bend your left arm behind your back. Raise your right arm, bend it at the elbow and attempt to clasp your fingertips together behind your back. Now try this exercise with the other side — you will probably find that you have one shoulder that is more flexible than the other. ULTIMATE ACHIEVEMENT: CLASPING FINGERTIPS OF BOTH HANDS BEHIND YOUR BACK ON EITHER SIDE

SO HOW ARE YOU DOING?

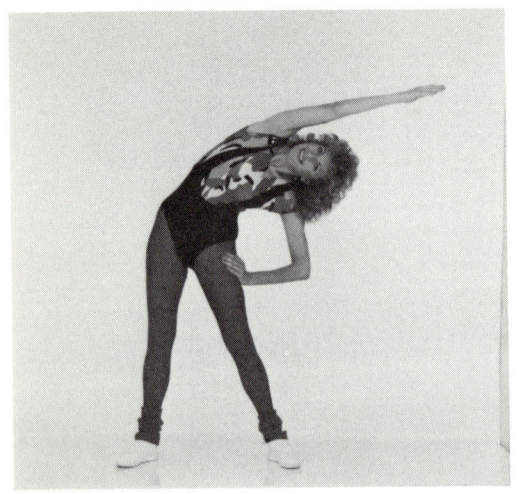

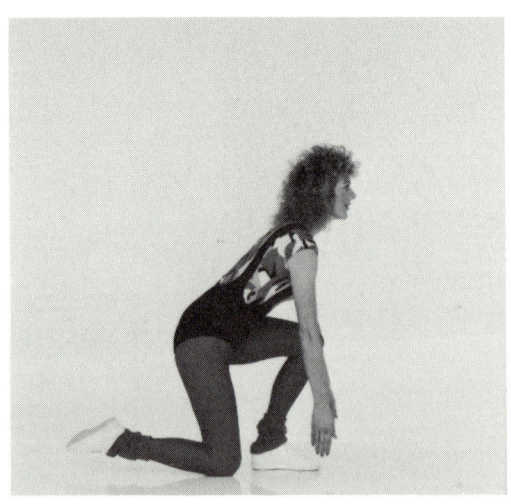

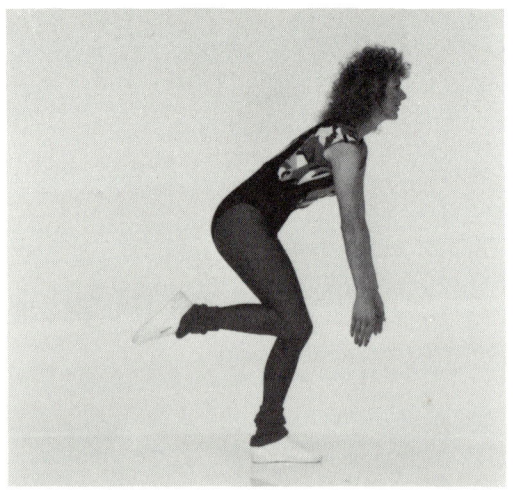

TORSO STRETCH
With your feet and legs a comfortable distance apart, raise your left arm and place your right hand on the top of your right thigh. Lean directly to your right side. Centralize and repeat, changing sides. Check your position — with *any* waist exercise you should rise out of the hips before leaning. Also, there should be no tilting backwards or forwards. ULTIMATE ACHIEVEMENT: REACHING OVER TO A NINETY DEGREE ANGLE ON BOTH SIDES

ULTIMATE THIGH TEST
Kneel on your right knee, lean forward and upright. Raise the toes of your right foot off the ground. →

Keeping your left foot flat on the floor, and *without* your right foot touching the ground, stand up. It helps to lean forward, and swinging the arms behind and then forward as you stand up gives you added impetus. Try the other leg. You will find a definite difference in strength between your left and right thighs.
ULTIMATE ACHIEVEMENT: TO STAND UP WITH EASE, WITHOUT LEANING FORWARD, ON *BOTH* LEGS

SO HOW ARE YOU DOING?

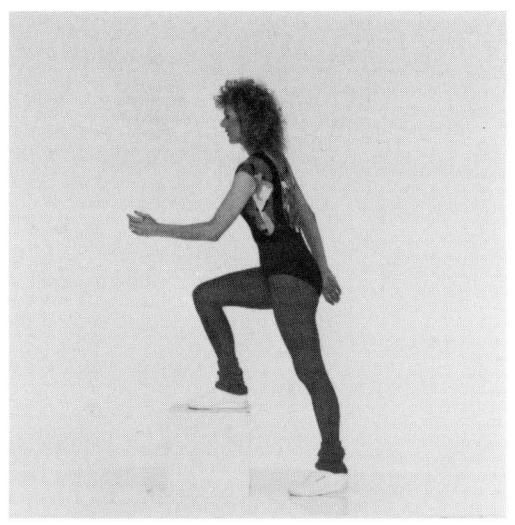 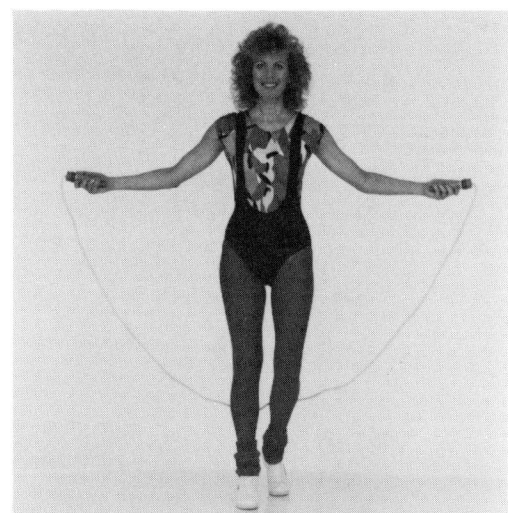 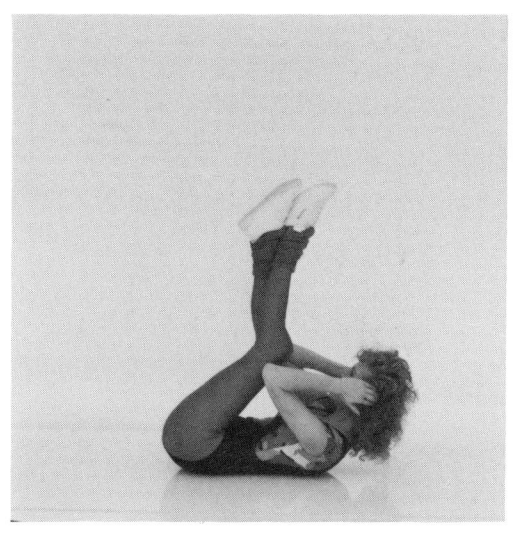

STAMINA
Using a steep stair or solid box, step up with your right, then your left foot, and down right, down left. Keep it rhythmical and as you get fitter increase the pace. ULTIMATE ACHIEVEMENT: TO CONTINUE THIS TEST FOR ONE FULL MINUTE AND AIM TO EXTEND THE LENGTH OF TIME EACH TIME YOU TEST YOURSELF

AEROBIC
With a skipping rope, lightly skip at a fast pace. You can keep yourself entertained by crossing your skipping rope and changing footwork. ULTIMATE ACHIEVEMENT: TO SKIP FOR 4–5 MINUTES – AND WANT TO DO MORE!

TUMMY STRENGTH
Lying on your back, lightly place your hands at the side of your head and cross your legs in the air at the ankles. Keep your head off the ground at all times. In a small rocking motion, reach forward, elbows touching knees (or beyond) and back. Exhale as you touch your knees. ULTIMATE ACHIEVEMENT: 50+

Once you have attained these ultimate achievement figures, don't stop – they are but guidelines!

Progress Chart

Test yourself every month and complete this chart.

	JUL	AUG	SEPT	OCT	NOV	DEC
THIGH HOLD Time yourself. How long can you comfortably hold this exercise? a) feet in b) feet out						
HIGH MARCHING How many can you do?						
SHOULDER SUPPLENESS Fill in when your fingertips are: a) nearly touching b) touching c) firmly grasping – both sides						
TORSO STRETCH						
ULTIMATE THIGH TEST Fill in when you can rise up: a) with difficulty b) to a standing position c) without leaning forward						
STAMINA How long can you continuously step up and down?						
AEROBIC How long can you skip? Either count or time yourself						
TUMMY How many can you do?